To My Family

To My Family

Michael Alan Seliner

ISBN: 1533583684
ISBN 13: 9781533583680
Library of Congress Control Number: 2016909192
CreateSpace Independent Publishing Platform
North Charleston, South Carolina

Contents

Acknowledgments

To Mom, Dad, Debbie, Vincent, Nathan, and Grace Jane:

I have written this book for the love of each of you as much as for the love of myself. I have grown and matured through the years as I desperately tried to fight a chronic disease that all but stole every aspect of my life except my love for you.

If for no other reason, it is for the sake of my sanity that I try to reconcile myself to a disease that has transformed me both physically and mentally.

I grew up believing in an all-knowing and all-loving God. For this gift, I have my parents to thank. Since the onset of this disease some twenty-five years ago, my will has been tested to its fullest and has even been shattered at times. I have grown older now and am reflecting on my life, and I once again believe and trust in the all-knowing and all-loving God whom I mistakenly believed had forsaken me.

To my family, I beg your forgiveness for the things you may have witnessed and heard. There is no going back; the arrow of time only points forward. Please know how painfully deep my love runs for each of you and that this book would not have been possible without you by my side, as I simply would not have had the will to write it. To my friends and those who have loved and supported me despite my rejections, know that I have always loved you; I offer no excuses.

To Michelle, note that all you have done has not been lost on me; I will always remember.

To my God, I understand now that You have never forsaken me, that when there was only one set of footprints in the earth below me, they belonged to You as You carried me through the difficult times. I am forever grateful for Your love and the life that You have breathed into me, not once but twice. I beg of You to not judge me too harshly—I have done only the best I can.

Love always and forever,
Your son, your father, your brother

A Fool's Errand

April 5, 2008.

I awoke early in the morning slumped over the same desk that I had passed out at the night before. This was an idiotic maneuver on my part as I was shaking from the cold of the morning air; the furnace had yet to kick on. I got up gingerly and walked to the bedroom, where I climbed into our empty king-size bed and slipped under the goose-down comforter.

A cramping and stiff neck forced me to take a dose of muscle relaxer—Zanaflex, to be exact. That's one drug I would reject under any other circumstance as it inevitably knocked me out within thirty minutes of ingestion and left me with memories of horrible nightmares—just another side effect of just another drug in my repertoire of many.

I heard my family downstairs and decided to make my way down. I knew that medication-induced sleep would soon be on its way. I grabbed the comforter, threw it over my back, and headed down.

"When did you decide to finally wake up?" Michelle asked in a tone that demanded an answer.

"What's that supposed to mean? It's eight o'clock," I replied.

"Mean? It means that more than half the time you walk around here in an absolute haze, paying attention to absolutely nothing except for your work and that damn computer. The times that you do take a break, it's like you're Rip Van Winkle, but the fable's true for you, Michael. Jesus, I can't even get you to sit down at the table and have a meal with us, with your own children. That's what I mean," she replied in an even harsher tone. She seemed to be trying her best to drag me into a conversation that I simply would have no part of. The conversation was always one-sided and recursive; therefore it was simply useless, to put it mildly.

This is going to be a wonderful weekend, I thought, and it was only Saturday morning.

Groundhog Day, I thought as I stared straight through her. Was she aware that I was not paying attention to her or even looking at her? *What was that giant groundhog's name in that movie? Bill something or other, or was that Bill Murray that I was thinking of? Christ, why can't I remember this? Punxsutawney Phil! Yep, that was his name, and Bill Murray called him a rat—absolutely hilarious.*

That's what I was—a groundhog (not a rat) that saw my own shadow every time I emerged from my den of ignorance, which was pretty nicely decorated.

She's right, I thought as I took a few backward steps away from her, avoiding yet another calamitous attempt at a conversation toward some sort of reconciliation, a final solution for an issue that seemed impossible to solve or even tack down. Why was every conversation she initiated about fixing me in some manner? I waited for her to turn around and not see me walk out of the room with my back toward her.

There was comfort in the haze though, comfort in seeing my shadow and keeping myself locked up in my warm, comfortable den. Sometimes ignorance really was bliss, but the life I was living was a lie, and my fate was to not discover this fact until it was too late. How much time was I wasting pretending that what I did for a living and the money I made was somehow more of a measure of a man, a measure of my own self-worth, than the love I had for my family or for myself? I was on a fool's errand, racing toward the finish line of life, and yet I wasn't even aware of it.

I made eye contact with my eldest son, Vincent, as I turned around and walked out of the kitchen. He shrugged his shoulders and started giggling as his mother continued talking. *Stop and smell the roses*, I thought. Perhaps the situation deserved some levity. Or perhaps the situation wasn't all that funny but sad instead.

DEPARTURE

March 9, 2007.

"Hi, Michael. My name's Bob. Come on in and make yourself comfortable."

Man, how I would have loved to lie down and stretch out on one of those couches and bury my head among the many decorative pillows. I was sure I could have been asleep within fifteen minutes, even with the lights on. I noticed the little white-noise machine that sat near the doorway, ensuring that disturbances were kept to a minimum. It looked like a white miniature shelf speaker.

Was this the look, the feel that Bob was going for? One immensely oversize leather couch, one decent-size leather love seat, one plush, oversize leather recliner with a rocking feature, a glass coffee table, an ornate throw rug, a ceiling fan, and one laminated wood desk that could have sat two people but was apparently reserved for Bob alone. That desk had nothing on it besides Bob's monthly calendar, a professionally taken photograph of him and his family, and a placard with his name and title neatly stenciled into the woodwork. However, I imagined that his desk drawers were filled with junk and miscellaneous knickknacks that really had no other place to go besides the garbage can, stuff that he had collected over the years that represented the juxtaposition of what the eyes could see.

The office was neatly decorated just enough to make one feel comfortable, and it was quite large, probably twice the size of my master bedroom.

To the left of Bob's enormous desk sat a floor-to-ceiling bookshelf that held not just books but also ornaments that appeared to be collected from either Africa or Pier 1 Imports. I had seen pictures of similar items from Africa, but Bob didn't seem like the type of person who visited there too often; Pier 1 suited him better than big-game hunting.

Bob apparently liked to read, as in a lot, or at least give the impression that he did. Outside of this study, I had never seen such a large personal collection of books. Some of them, I noticed, had been read recently, as they were not placed neatly back in their appropriate slots, and the dust that had once covered the shelves was missing. They were placed on their sides, facedown, as if they had been dropped there in a hurried fashion prior to someone entering his office.

I thought it odd, however, the lack of plaques that one usually finds within the office of such a well-studied man. Maybe he didn't have any, which I doubted, or maybe he didn't believe in keeping them out as part of his office decor. I'll never know the answer to this question though as I never asked it. I knew Bob, however, would have plenty of questions for me.

Bob sat down in his old, worn desk chair, which also had a swivel and recline feature that he was apparently quite fond of. He had even gone so far as to decorate it with a plush, blue-corduroy seat pad and a set of wooden back beads that made noise every time he moved around in that old chair. The chair itself made noises every time it moved around, for that matter.

He grabbed his leather-bound legal notebook, pulled out a gold-plated pen from his shirt pocket—a Cross pen, I noticed (must have been a gift)—pushed his glasses up the bridge of his nose, and stared at me. Bob wore oversize square bifocal glasses that didn't quite fit his face. He also wore a chain on the earpieces, as if he were worried that the glasses would somehow blow off. They were bifocals, after all, so what was the point of constantly taking them on and off?

He made a single entry in his notebook before he began to speak—it had to be the date and time. From all outward appearances, Bob seemed to be a rather neat fellow who appreciated his space appearing neat to others also. I believe that he took some pride in the fact that he could check off at least one item in his job description that he was doing well—ensuring that his visitors noted his neatness and appreciated it. If I had been asked to do a postvisit survey, I would have given him high marks in this area.

Bob was probably about my age, maybe a little older now that I noticed his graying hair and crow's feet, along with the many creases in his forehead. I could only begin to imagine the stories that were told in this room that put those creases in Bob's forehead over years of him diligently performing his job. They didn't come from conversations involving happiness or joy. They came from years of listening to conversations that caused him great consternation and constant frowning. How many times over the years had he listened to the same story being told by different people? How many times had he given out the same advice to different people and charged the same amount of money?

I couldn't help but wonder what exactly Bob's motivation was. There had to be a certain amount of boredom inherent in his job. Did he have a true interest in helping people, or was it all about getting through that next session and cashing that next check? Honestly, I wasn't too concerned about that. I had a story to tell, like everyone else, and I wanted someone to listen to it—check that, I *needed* someone to listen to it. Was I about to tell Bob the same old crappy story that he had heard time and again? Was that little voice in his head about to start praying, "Please, God, not again"? Whether Bob truly cared, I'll never know, and that's just one more detail that I'll have to live without.

"So how can I help you today, Michael?" Bob asked. "By the way, do you prefer Michael or Mike?"

I can't count the number of times I've been asked that question. Well, I probably could if I had properly kept track of the number of hospital visits I had over the years, but it's too late for that now. *You're starting off on the wrong foot, Bob,* I thought. *Is that supposed to be the politically correct way of asking, or is it just an icebreaker? Hell, who gives a shit what you call me, Bob?* That's what I was thinking of saying, anyway; my sense of humor is pretty dry, but I don't think Bob would have appreciated that remark too much.

"Mike's fine," I replied.

Where do I start? After all, I had a lot to talk about, and my issues were not going to be resolved within the next hour. *"Bob, I'm not quite sure how to put this, but there's a fucking freight train coming down the tunnel, and you better get the hell off the tracks."* No, I shouldn't start things off that way. Let's try the politically correct way, the boring way.

"Bob, I first want to ensure that we have some ground rules in place, if you will, that we both agree to," I said.

"OK—I'm not quite sure what that means. Maybe you can elaborate on that point for me, please," he replied.

"I'm not quite sure how to word this, but I want to know what things I may say that will set off alarm bells in your mind, so to speak. For example, if I were to tell you that I am addicted to painkillers and have a private stash at my home and am selling them, what would you be legally bound to do?" I asked.

"OK, I see. You want to know some hypothetical scenarios in which I would be obligated to report to the police or authorities, correct?" he said.

"Hypothetical, exactly, and don't get me wrong—I was once placed in a very awkward situation—back-stabbed, you might say—in my not-too-distant past by a fucking social worker, and I do not wish to have a repeat."

"Well, the best I can do is to give you some examples of things that if you were to divulge to me, I would be legally obligated to report to authorities. Otherwise I would tell you let's just cross those bridges if and when we get to them, OK?" he said.

I nodded my head in agreement and listened as Bob continued on about suicidal tendencies (great band), harming others, threatening him, drugs, and so on. Bob painted a pretty good picture of the things that could and could not be said within the boundaries of those four walls. I had found a safe house, insulated in thick, cold steel plate—a bomb shelter of sorts. It was a little bothersome and quite obvious, however, that Bob had found my question somewhat concerning and confusing at the same time. It was another example of a topic that put yet another wrinkle in his forehead.

I would say that overall things didn't get off to a good start with Bob. I knew I would have to work at it a bit to make Bob feel more comfortable and get on with the business of helping me with my needs. Why did I find psychologists and social workers to be like Play-Doh in my hands? Was it concerning that I found some pleasure in molding them how I wanted? Perhaps the better question was, why was I in the position of seeing so many of these types of therapists in the first place?

"So have I answered your questions or concerns, Mike?" he asked.

"Yes, thank you for taking the time to explain that to me," I replied.

"That's quite all right, but I have to admit that I've never been asked those questions before. You must have given this meeting quite a bit of thought prior to today. Do you feel comfortable enough to move on now?" Bob asked.

"Sure," I replied. I should've asked Bob the same question. Was Bob ready to hear what I was about to tell him? Was he ready to heal me? Could he heal me? I knew that only time would tell. For all I knew, this session might be the first and the last, the alpha and the omega.

"Can you tell me the reason why you sought the help of a psychologist?" he asked.

"Well, I recently changed insurance companies, and with that move, I had to change several of my regular doctors. One of those doctors was my psychiatrist, Dr. Zhiad. I had an appointment with him about a week ago, and it was mainly to refill my standing prescriptions of Pristiq and Abilify. However, once I started talking with him, I realized that maybe it would be a good idea to ask him if there were newer or better drugs on the market besides those as I have been feeling kind of blue, a little erratic, not so much myself as of late.

"Dr. Zhiad decided to add ten milligrams of Abilify to my Pristiq as it has shown relatively quick success in helping other drugs such as antidepressants work more effectively. He also mentioned that drugs are not always the answer and that he thought that I would benefit from some sort of therapy. My PCP actually recommended you," I said.

"Oh, yeah? Who's your PCP?" he asked.

"Dr. Mason," I replied.

"Oh, yeah, he and I go way back. Funny though, I haven't heard his name mentioned lately," he said. Another wrinkle on his forehead was forming as he spoke. He was obviously bothered by the fact that he hadn't heard from his old friend Dr. Mason in quite some time. "How's he doing?" he asked.

"He's doing great. I understand he has a family of three now, and his business couldn't be doing better. You know as well as I that he is a personable individual," I said.

Bob was obviously happy not just to hear that Dr. Mason was doing well but to hear his name again at all, judging by the big-ass grin on his face. Kind of strange, I remember thinking.

"Well, Mike, I can tell you that your psychiatrist is an intelligent individual. Drugs are not the answer to everything, and in your case, they don't seem to be helping all that much, which may be attributed to the MS."

Strange…when did I mention that I have MS? No, I'm quite sure that I didn't. Where the hell did he get that from? Oh, those goddamn forms. Jesus, I swear there had to be five or six pages of questions about everything from when I first had sex to whether I ever thought about killing myself. There was a little box at the bottom of one of the forms under the heading "Medical Conditions" labeled "Other." Just thinking about it made me want to puke all over Bob's floor. This wasn't just an "Other" topic—MS was the singularity that caused the Big Bang for me.

"It also seems to me that you do have some things on your mind that you need to talk about, and I think that's the key, for now anyway. You just need to talk these things through," Bob replied. "If you don't mind, Mike, I like to try to gather a broader picture of the clients that I work with, and what that usually entails is starting from the beginning, if you will. Sound OK?" he asked.

"Sure, fire away," I said.

"So if you don't mind me asking, why are you in a wheelchair?" he asked.

I have to admit, I was somewhat flabbergasted by the question and the arrogant boldness of this person to ask it. However, I'm a pretty straightforward guy, and I don't appreciate bullshit answers to valid questions. I guess what bothered me was whether it was a valid question or one of simple curiosity. I've put up with a lot of shit over the years since being diagnosed with MS, and while I don't feel that entitles me to anything special, I do believe that I am entitled to my privacy, especially given the fact that MS is such a privacy-invading disease to begin with.

Let's face it, it's only human nature to take a second look at someone using an assistive device such as a cane, walker, or wheelchair; throw in a judgment about that person, and suddenly you're a bigot. When I'm out in public, I may give someone in a wheelchair a second look if for no other reason than to check out his or her ride. Levity is always the key in a situation such as this, but I could find nothing in his question besides odd curiosity. There was no follow-up—he just buried the lead and that was it.

I have an extremely short fuse, and that fuse quickly ignites into rage, according to more than one therapist. That was one of the underlying reasons I was there talking with Bob. As luck would have it, Bob asked the one question that would spark the anger and quickly flame into rage. The rage inside me built to a crescendo, a beautiful, head-pounding grunge that I could hear blaring in my eardrums and nothing else. In that instant, I wanted nothing more than to take a running leap at Bob and sucker-punch him straight in the mouth, knocking a few of those beautiful, polished white teeth out. White turns to red in a flash flood of blood; broken teeth lie strewn across Bob's lap. Was this the answer he was looking for? I had to keep my monster under wraps.

Rage, however, is the antithesis of what the word itself implies: a sheep in wolf's clothing. Any therapist worth his or her degree can tell you that at the heart of rage is fear, words that are easily spoken but difficult to accurately define, even by the finest wordsmiths. I am fearful, very fearful, but that does not preclude me from the raw feeling of rage itself and what it may bring about. Regardless of exactly what the meds I am on are supposed to prevent, I know all too well what happens to me and what I am capable of not only feeling but *doing*. For me, this is where the fear steps in.

As I thought about Bob's question, I had to consider his reason for asking it. Maybe he did have a valid reason. Maybe he knew someone in a wheelchair, maybe a best friend, maybe a family member. Maybe he just wanted to see what my reaction would be. Maybe I didn't give a shit. Maybe, just maybe all that junk from Africa and all those books on his bookshelves were nothing but a bunch of decorative crap.

I found myself in a conundrum. Already Bob was getting the upper hand on me, and this simply wasn't to be. No, I needed to mold this giant hunk of Play-Doh back into place. I needed to play it cool, calm, and collected. I needed to take it down a notch. This was not who I wanted to be any longer. The word "rebel" was losing its meaning for me.

I knew one thing for sure—I had already decided that I liked Bob, but most importantly, I had not grown to trust Bob yet. He deserved an answer, and I had to trust him if he was ever going to be able to help me. "Bob, I have a simple question for you first." Ah, dammit, here we go—Schrödinger's cat all over again! I couldn't leave well enough alone. Why? "Bob, I'm curious to know where you got all of those knickknacks that you have on your bookshelves. It looks like they came from Africa. Did they?" I asked. I had a game plan in mind, and that was that I wanted to find out whether Bob was ready to show his hand. If not, then I would simply find myself a new therapist. If so, then I would continue and give him the answer.

"No, they're not from Africa. They're actually from Central America, and I certainly didn't travel there. I have a friend who travels there quite a bit for work, and he purchased them for me as gifts. Apparently he found out that I was fond of the first one he gave me and—well, let's just say that the gifts keep coming."

There you have it, plain and simple: the truth isn't that hard to speak. Only when we have spun a web of lies is there no going back, no undoing the lies. The truth will set you free, Bob, and lies will damn you to hell. My mind pulled the short straw to hell a long time ago, second only to my body, and I find it outrageous.

"I'm in a wheelchair, Bob, because I have a disease, MS, and have lost the use of my legs. By the way, you said you wanted to start from the beginning. You're kind of starting at the end," I told him. "Do you not wish to talk about the disease itself, Bob?" Just one more stab in the back before moving on. *Stupid is as stupid does*, I thought. *Isn't that a quote from a movie? Yes, I believe it's from* Forrest Gump.

As I was sitting there having a ridiculous conversation with myself, I looked down from the ceiling and saw that Bob was still sitting there, acting as if he were waiting to hear an answer from me when he was the one who owed me an answer.

"No, nothing against you, Mike. I feel that we'll talk about it at some point, but there're other things in your life that occurred way before your being diagnosed with this disease. I'd like to talk about those things first," he said.

OK, I thought. *Didn't I just say that to him? Anyway, if Bob wants the whole nine yards, then that's what I'll give him, as crazy as some of the stuff may sound. I'll let Bob Gump drive this Winnebago for now.*

ADOPTION

April 2, 1978.

"I love you." Those three simple words can have such a profound impact on a person, especially a child. I have tried over and over to remember the first time that I heard these words spoken by either of my parents, but each time I have failed. Not because they never spoke these words but because of a memory lock that I lost the key to a long time ago in the darkness where memories should lie; a room with keys hanging from the ceiling. How long does it take to utter these simple words? How many times must they have been uttered to me as a child?

My mother was sitting on my father's side of their king-size bed, perfectly calm, arms open, accepting me into her loving embrace as she hugged me tightly. She motioned for me to sit down beside her, and I nervously asked what she wanted to talk about. I had only been given short notice that she wanted to speak with me, but I didn't know what about. There was an open window next to the bed, and a slight breeze made its way into the house as it gently ruffled the curtain sheers, which caressed the ornate ceramic lamp that sat atop the white wooden nightstand. There was a distinctive sound that I had become accustomed to of the wind blowing through the screen; a thunderstorm was looming, and while I could not yet hear the boom of thunder, I could see flashes of lightning against a darkened backdrop of rolling clouds.

The room was dimly lit, with the only light coming from that single bedroom window. The light was further darkened by an outdoor aluminum window overhang that helped block out the sunlight during the hotter months of summer. I could tell that it was about to rain as the smell of ozone permeated the room, and the humidity was on the climb. It was peaceful, and if left to my own devices, I would have quickly fallen asleep.

I hugged my mother, responding back in kind. My love for her ran deep; it was unshakable, and I trusted her fully. She spoke gently, alerting me to the fact that what she was about to say was somehow important. Perhaps she did not want my sister or father to hear what she was about to tell me, though I could come up with no good reason why. My mother did not believe in keeping secrets, and most of all, she did not believe in telling lies of any sort. This was her modus operandi, her main beliefs in life that I grew up with.

My mother was strong at heart, and she stared me directly in the eyes when she said that she had something very important to tell me and asked that I give her my full attention. I had never seen tears in her eyes before let alone seen her cry; this was one of those moments.

"What's wrong, Mom?" I asked.

She held on to my hands tightly, staring deeply into my eyes. I could not look away but became fidgety.

"Sometimes in life, Michael, mothers and fathers cannot take proper care of their children. Sometimes mothers get very sick, sometimes they do not have the money they need to raise their children, and sometimes they are too young to have children, but one thing to remember is that mothers and fathers always love their children. Do you understand?" she asked.

"Yes, Mom," I replied.

Her hands now drew away from mine, and she clasped them over her face and began to gently cry.

I grabbed her hands away from her face. I was scared, I was panicked, and I didn't understand the situation. There was a barely noticeable crackle in my voice. "What is wrong, Mom? Why are you crying?"

"Michael, do you know what being adopted means? Have you ever heard the term?" she asked.

"No," I replied.

With her composure regained, she began to tell me a secret that had been kept perfectly quiet for the past eleven years. The air within this room where this secret had been kept was stagnant and had a pungent odor. "When you were a baby, you had another mother, a biological mother, your birth mother, and you also had another father, a biological father," she began. "Your biological mother was very young, about fifteen, and your biological father was about sixteen, and neither of them was able to take proper care of you at that young of an age. When your father and I first saw you, we fell in love with you, honey."

I couldn't understand. What was she talking about?

The confusion must have been easy for her to read on my face. Again, she squeezed me tightly and gently cried over my shoulder.

I pushed her back to look into her eyes again. I told her that I didn't understand what she was saying. "Are you and Dad leaving me?" I asked. The very thought made me shudder in fear.

"No, no, no, never ever would we leave you, honey. This is what adoption is; this is what adoption means," she explained. "This is what makes you so special. It means that you have a mother who gave birth to you, who loved you very much but was too young to take care of you. But you have family that loves you very much now, your father and me. We adopted you and your sister as our own children. You are a very special person, Michael, and we will always love you," she said.

I understood. It was strange, though—I had no questions, nothing to ask, nothing to add. My mother had put all the pieces to the puzzle very neatly together, and I liked the picture she created.

The carpet in her bedroom was a deep, plush red with a worn-down area close to the closet where my father got dressed for work every morning. I stared at this area for some time, emotionless, shoulders slumped, thinking. I pictured my father pacing back and forth in front of the closet as he picked out his clothes and got dressed for work every morning.

My mother interrupted my daydreaming and asked if I wanted to be alone.

I hugged her and said, "You're my mother, Mom. You have always been my mother."

She cried and I hugged her; it upset me immensely to see her cry, and I tried as hard as I could to console her.

My father was not in the bedroom that day; that fact was not lost on me. He was not in attendance for what was probably the most important discussion of his life. Why? Was he worried about the possibility of rejection from me? Had I failed him in some manner? As I made my way back to my bedroom, down the end of the hallway, I glimpsed him sitting in his recliner in the family room around the corner. He was smoking a cigarette and watching the television set; there was a special nervousness about his actions.

As I quietly opened the door to my bedroom, I paused for a moment and looked back over my shoulder at him one last time. He sat there, staring intently at the television. *Maybe a newsworthy story is breaking; he is a news junkie*, I thought. His gaze never met mine as I looked at him briefly over my shoulder, and he remained silent. I went into my room, turned around, and gently shut the door, releasing the knob slowly so as not to make a noise. I was still staring at him through the door, questioning why. Why did my father have nothing to say to me? Was this just another day to him? Was he staring back at me through my closed door?

I had felt uplifted by the conversation with my mother, but now I simply felt nothing. Who was this man I called father? Was there some pain associated with the situation that was too great for him to bear? Was he concerned about letting his emotions show? Did he love me as much as my mother did? I truly could not answer that question, and it still eludes me today on some level.

Years passed, and when I was sixteen, I came to understand why my father was not in the room with us that day. I never heard it spoken from his lips, but this was my interpretation as told to me by my mother. Maybe my interpretation is just an opinion, one of many that could have been formulated that day.

Most couples adopt children based on only a handful of reasons. Some couples' love for children is so great that they wish to share it with others who are less fortunate, such as children who would not otherwise be adopted due to a variety of unfortunate issues. Others may not be able to have children of their own due to a variety of issues such as sterility. As it turned out, this was the issue that prevented my father from having children. Like I said, my mother gave a reason—not the reason for my father not being there that day for what would turn out to be the biggest day of my life. Sterility in and of itself cannot be labeled as the reason for not wanting to attend this special conversation; it was simply an excuse. I felt sorry for him.

DEBRA

Born October 3, 1970, Debbie Lynn Seliner was three
years and four days younger than me. She was my
sister. "Debra," as she demanded to be called, was even
more different from our family than I had already begun
to understand. I was the only one in the family who got
away with calling her Debbie She had made herself an
outcast; that was of no one's doing but her own.

I could hear her grab hold of the doorknob to my
parent's bedroom to open the door. As one door opened,
another was about to close. I had already realized that
her world was about to come crashing down around her.
I did not take this matter lightly as I cared immensely
for my younger sister and had tried hard to protect her
from things that would cause her more grief. This was
one case where I had no say, where my lips were sewn
shut, where my mouth suddenly became dry as cotton.
The door shut, and I heard her lay down on the bed
next to my mother. An odd thought, but I wondered if

my mother would ask her to please sit up during their conversation or if she would let her lie down. Either way, I knew Debbie would be standing by the end of the conversation, perhaps even ready to run out of the room and out of the house altogether.

I felt sorry for my mother because I was concerned that Debbie might deeply wound her with a few sharp, well-placed words from which she might not be able to recover.

Debbie was a tomboy plain and simple. Her personality was in your face, and she could strike like a cobra at any time. She could be your best friend one minute and your worst enemy the next. She lived in the moment, at least when she was high. The lows seem to be brought on by nothing in particular, and when she was experiencing a low moment, you were like the rat running across the snake's path.

Plain and simple, Debbie was a tomboy with a time bomb, and that time bomb had a technical name: bipolar disorder, a diagnosis that I would come to learn about from my mother during my first year of college. It was a diagnosis that I did not understand all too well, but I did understand and suffer from its side effects firsthand. A massive black hole, nothing escaped Debbie's depressive episodes, not even one's own emotions. Thinking back on it now, I'm quite sure that militaries of the 1970s and

1980s tried their best to conjure up a nerve agent in order to deploy bipolar disorder to the battlefield. What a perfect weapon that would've made to cripple the opponent.

Debbie didn't drink alcohol at all from what I remember, not even a beer with the boys so to speak as she grew older. Her manic episodes could keep her sky-high for months on end. There simply was no street-drug substitute. She liked to stay indoors most of the time with her cats and watch old black-and-white movies on a TV that my parents had let go years prior, especially ones starring Vincent Price, who was born in St. Louis. I guess you could call them horror movies for the time they were shot in.

She did have one vice, however, and that was smoking. As soon as my parents were tired of fighting with her over her young age, she officially began smoking at the age of fifteen. I'm not exactly sure who bought the cigarettes for her, and had I found out, I'm sure I would've done more than a little damage to him or her.

The cigarettes she smoked were about the skinniest things that I had ever seen. I don't remember what they were called, but I do remember seeing a commercial one time for Virginia Slims, and her cigarettes were about half the diameter of those. They weren't tobacco-colored either; they were white with a butterfly on the outside of the box. Strange, however, I remember my father being the biggest proponent of her smoking. I used to think what a hypocrite he was for even bringing it up in the first place; after all, he was a chain-smoker himself, probably three packs per day. The cigarettes were definitely a vice to help get her through the depressive episodes. Pharmaceuticals seemed to have little effect, and she often refused to take them.

I could hear from my room, behind closed doors and down the hallway, my sister and my mother having the same conversation that I just had. I had wondered why my mother didn't have the same conversation with both Debbie and I at the same time. The answer eluded me.

A sudden clap of thunder as lightning struck the nearby TV station tower caught me off guard and interrupted my thoughts. I could hear my father, still sitting in his recliner, now watching nothing but white noise on his television, cussing at the storm and sucking down a cigarette. He could put down a cigarette in two drags. Two drags meant a great deal of aggravation, irritation, a fatal myocardial infarction waiting to strike at any moment. No, there was no missing the fact that this was a tense moment for my father, a moment that had most likely been building toward a crescendo for quite some time now. How long had it been? Who knows for certain, but reflecting back now, I know it had been on his mind for quite some time. My father, like most men, was a procrastinator, and it was apparent to me that he had been procrastinating over having this conversation.

I knew that the conversation with my mom and sister would not go over well. I don't know why exactly, call it intuition, but in any event it would turn out to be her new reality. This fact upset me, but I knew that there was nothing that I could do or say that would make any difference. Debra had to let things play out in her mind—it had always been that way no matter how small the detail. Her mind was forever stuck in minutia. I never faulted her for her actions. That was simply who she was, right?

I sat on the floor next to the windowsill in my room. The window was wide open, and I could see the dust and dirt piled up on the sill and knew that it would take a good amount of paper towels and glass cleaner to clean up the mess. I also knew that I would be the one cleaning it up. It was springtime, and it was evident that the window had not been opened in quite some time. Without the window open, it would have been difficult to see clearly through the glass as it too was covered with dirt and water stains.

It was a comfortable spring afternoon now that the thunderstorm had passed, and I could feel the breeze making its way under my door and escaping through the window to the outdoors. I could smell spring in the air; I paused at the scent of the flowers coming from outside my parents' bedroom window. I heard my friends playing soccer down the street and laughing. I longed to be outdoors with my friends, to escape this situation that did not seem real to me. I wasn't being punished and could probably go outside on my own, but I wouldn't do so without asking my father's permission, but I did not want to speak with him. I decided it would be best to wait it out, wait for the conversation between parent and daughter to come to an end. How long was I speaking with my mother for? Maybe two hours? I grabbed a pillow off my bed and placed it on the carpeting under my head, staring up at the ceiling.

My entire ceiling was decorated with a collage of old Dairy Queen window posters I had obtained from the local store I frequented just prior to it going out of business. Hot fudge sundaes, banana splits, dilly bars, parfaits, malts, and shakes of all flavors. I'm sure I had the full collection up there on my ceiling. I can't tell you why I decided to staple all of those posters to my ceiling, nor could I tell my parents, who didn't take too kindly to me redecorating my room that way. I was just lucky that they didn't make me take them all down, but then they knew that they would have to stucco over all the holes in the ceiling from the staples.

My eyelids became heavy. With the slow approach of sunset came daydreaming of what had just transpired, when there was a sudden light knock at my door. It was Debbie asking if she could come in. Debbie always respected my privacy; there was no need for locked doors in the house. I knew what was coming, and I guess in the back of my mind somewhere, I was already searching for ways to console her. I knew that she would be upset and looking for answers that I too probably lacked. By the time I got to the door, I heard the whispered panic in her voice, her hurried rush to get inside my room, a safe haven of sorts where she could avoid my father, who still sat stoically in the family room staring at the television.

Time passed. This was the cooling-off period, I thought; a time for each of us to reflect on the major life change that had just transpired. She sat at the foot of my bed with her elbows on her knees and her hands on her face. I sat on the floor below my window with my back to the wall and my arms hanging over my knees. I felt the coolness of that early spring twilight penetrating the wall and chilling my back. The light breeze felt good and refreshing, though maybe a bit chilly to my sister; I didn't ask. I looked up at her, and she sat there with her legs crossed, quietly hunched over, hugging a pillow with her chin buried in it. She lifted her head as if to talk to me but instead only stared outside the window above my head. Debbie would initiate the conversation when she was ready. Time stood still.

My sister was beautiful, and it was at that moment that I realized what her biological mother must have looked like. Years later when I had children of my own, I came to realize what my parents must have looked like. This is all I had, a glimpse into a different path of life that might have been. I've held onto it for whatever the reason.

There was little light in my room now. What was left of the sunlight outside reflected onto the walls of my room and cast shadows all about. There was some comfort in the darkness, not so much for me but for my sister. I left the room light off. It had always been this way with her, and I never understood the real reason why until my teenage years. This, however, was not to be the topic of discussion this late afternoon. She need-ed to work out what had just transpired, and my own thoughts didn't matter.

She began to talk in a quiet tone at first. "Do you know what Mom just told me?" she asked. *Mom.* She had used the one word already that I figured she would never use again, a telling note for me to remember for future reference. My mother told me beforehand that she was going to talk with Debbie, so I knew this con-versation was coming and it would be with me, no one else. I knew I would be cheated out of the time alone that I required to process and neatly file this information or at least give to my assistant to take care of. "Just file it under *A* for adoption, please," I said out loud. After all, that's pretty much how it works, isn't it?

I knew that above all, my sister would require the most help getting through this. I also knew that, on some level, my mother expected me to help Debbie understand. My mother knew that my sister and I had a special and different type of relationship than most brothers and sisters. Debbie never had been and never would be part of the family unit, and as hard as my parents tried to get her to fit in, they failed time and again. Debbie knew that I accepted her for who she was, but then again, my parents had to be parents. This truly was the only key to unlocking my sister's mind, and though it was a simple key, it was one that few could understand. Explaining this to others was like asking them to solve the Rubik's Cube on their first attempt; it was impossible for the majority of people.

For reasons I will never understand, Debbie had a certain amount of faith in me. Her trust in me was unwavering. I had given her my word once and had never broken it. Trust was the one bond that held us together.

My relationship with my sister was also sad on some level. I don't think I recognized it fully at the time, but it was. I had plenty of friends to talk with, friends to go out and have fun with as a typical child should. I also had my parents, both a mother and father who I could speak openly and truthfully with at any time (more so my mother). Management calls it an "open-door policy." That day I needed to play the role of both her boss and brother.

Debra was the polar opposite of me in every respect. She preferred the darkness while I preferred the light. She preferred the loneliness while I preferred friendships. My parents constantly encouraged me to help my sister with her problems as they began to realize that they lacked the ability to do so. This was no fault of theirs. There was a very complex relationship between the four of us, and in some manner, we needed to work together to become a single unit, to become a family. If that was at all possible, only time would tell.

The silence was suddenly broken, "What do you think about what Mom just told us?" she asked me. It was a loaded question that one could ponder for weeks, months, if not years before drawing even the slightest conclusion. Nonetheless, I knew that, for my sister, this question was one that needed to be answered immediately. I paused when our eyes met for the first time, and I noticed she was beginning to cry. I understood, probably as much as my mother now, how delicate the situation was. This was the type of question, the type of event that could change one's life in an instant, and for my sister, I believe it already had.

I trod lightly as we began to talk, noting that I did not take lightly this information that my parents had apparently carried on their shoulders for years and had just now come to light.

I mustered up the best response that an eleven-year-old could give her. "What does this change for us, Debbie?"

Fighting her way through her tears, she simply said, "I'm afraid."

"Afraid of what?" I asked.

"They're not even our real parents," she said.

"What do you mean they're not our real parents? They most certainly are," I replied. "They've been our real parents since birth. Just who do you think our parents really are?" I suddenly found myself on the defensive. I felt an anger growing inside me that was directly pointed at her like the tip of a dart. I wanted to throw that dart right at her forehead. Yep, fifty points for striking that half-inch diameter circle that would hopefully wake her up. Her comment hit me deep, and I suddenly felt cold and clammy, and my stomach grew upset. It was not something I wanted to possess or hear.

Memories started to trickle back. A black box in the back corner of my mind that my psyche had created years ago to protect me, which had been sitting un-disturbed and dusty for years now, had suddenly been busted open, not by anything my mother had said, but by what my sister had said. Darkness flowed over my eyes, and the lights dimmed even further. Was I about to pass out?

I understood the definition of adoption, and I guess I wanted to leave it at just that—a definition, a word without much meaning filed under *A*. My black-and-white mind was good at burying things, burying them so deep that sometimes I could not even find them. I think my mind was already at work trying desperately to construct a new black box for this overflow of infor-mation. Maybe another hour in my room alone pro-cessing the information and I would have been fine. I would never have to remember that conversation with my mother again. All would be fine.

She sat there now on the edge of my bed throwing one of my pillows at me. She was highly agitated; I could tell by the way her voice pitched upward when she was in deep distress or confronted with something she didn't wish to talk about. My daydreaming caused me to forget what her question was to me.

"Is that it? Is that all you have to say? Don't you feel like we've been living with strangers?" she said.

"Strangers?" I laughed out loud at that comment. How ludicrous, I thought. I asked my sister a simple yet poignant question. "Have you always loved Mom and Dad?"

She hesitated momentarily, and then responded, "Yes, but I love Mom more than him."

Him. Again, a single word that carried a lot of meaning and memories, both good and bad. How in the world does anyone deal with it, let alone respond to a comment like that about your own father? They don't, or at least an eleven-year-old boy does not. I stared past her, through her to be more precise, and simply said, "I'm sorry you feel that way, Debra. I don't."

"Michael, I love you, but we're not even really brother and sister—we're adopted."

Shock and anger had finally overcome me; the cobra had struck at me, but not before I grabbed its neck like a mongoose trying to choke the life out of it. I yelled at her at the top of my lungs, knowing that my parents could hear every word I screamed. "What the hell is the matter with you, Debra? Who the hell do you love?"

In sheer panic, she begged me to lower my voice, not wanting anyone to hear. She could barely maintain her breath now; she could barely speak to me.

"Debbie, do you love Mom now, right now, after having the conversation you just had with her?"

"Yes, I still love her very much, but I hate him. Jesus, Michael, he wasn't even in the room with her, with me. Has he even spoken to you?"

I didn't need to answer this question; it was redundant. What neither of us knew was why. Would his attendance have made the entire conversation easier or more difficult? I already knew the answer, but I decided to pose it to her, not as a question but more as a statement. "Debbie, you realize that they are our parents. They are the only thing that we have ever known. They have been there with us since birth. They have loved and cared for us since birth. You know Dad has problems dealing with emotional issues such as this and that will probably never change. In my mind, that is only further proof that nothing about this has changed. Please do not be angry with either of them."

Before leaving the room, Debbie responded by saying, "I cannot be angry at Mom at all. I love her very much, but I do not think that I can say the same about

Dad." She shut the door behind her, and I simply sat there on the floor staring at the closed door and imagining what my father must have been feeling. I listened intently but didn't hear any conversation between my parents. I don't know what I would have done if I had.

I pulled the cover from the end of my bed and over me and fell asleep on the floor crying quietly. My parents let me be; they were smart enough to know that I would come to them.

Another knock on my door woke me from my sleep. It was my sister again, and she was there to report that my mother and father were in their room talking, "whispering," as she called it. My sister's room was right next to my parents' room, and a tightly pressed ear against the cool wall could pick up just about any conversation. Although I was not desperate for any of the news that might come from their room, my sister was, so in order to try to somehow abate her fears, I followed her to her room where we could listen in private together.

Once there, we opened the door partway to make it seem as though we had left her room altogether. Then we hid in her closet with the bifold doors shut tight. As my father was hard of hearing from years of working at a machine shop, my mother had to speak up quite a bit in order for him to hear her. Fortunately for my sister and me, this made for easy listening to a conversation that would have otherwise been impossible to hear. We could hear my mother apparently trying to calm my father down by telling him that our conversations seem to have gone well and that no one had cried or become overly upset. I heard my father ask a question out of the blue that caught me off guard.

"Did either of them ask why I was not in the room with you?" It was the very question that I had so desperately wanted to ask my mother only hours before but did not have the nerve.

"No, Donald, neither of them asked where you were. Are you happy now?"

I could not tell by my mother's tone whether she was being sarcastic or not, which left me fidgeting around inside the closet, with my sister trying to get me to quiet down. An answer still eluded me. My sister had no questions, only doubt.

To My Mother…

Once there were two women
Who never knew each other.
One you do not remember,
The other you call mother.

Two different lives
Shaped to make you one.
One became your guiding star,
The other became your sun.

The first one gave you life,
The second taught you to live it.
The first gave you a need for love,
The second was there to give it.

One gave you a nationality.
The other gave you a name.
One gave you a talent.
The other gave you aim.

One gave you emotions.
The other calmed your fears.
One saw your first sweet smile.
The other dried your tears.

One sought for you a home
That she could not provide.
The other prayed for a child,
And her hope was not denied.

And now you ask me
Through your tears
The age-old question
Unanswered through the years.
Heredity or environment,
Which are you a
product of?

Neither, my darling,
Neither.
Just two kinds of love.

THERAPY 101

March 23, 2007.

By the time my first session came to an end, I'm sure Bob had quite the cramp in his hand from writing so feverishly. I had always wondered why therapists never used tape recorders in lieu of writing; maybe some did, or at least the ones that I saw in the movies did. Bob also never got into the habit of saying, "OK, our session has come to an end for the day." I had seen my fair share of therapists throughout my life, and Bob was starting to grow on me. I liked his quirkiness, his ability to put me at ease by asking simple questions like whether you wanted his ceiling fan on or off.

Bob was quite particular about his ceiling fan. He didn't need to tell me—I knew that he liked to have it on. Even when it was slightly cool outside, his office was warm, and Bob made a point to talk about how he already had to turn the air conditioner on inside his office in early spring. The architect of the building had made a fatal design flaw and must've been a real dumb shit to the dismay of the HVAC engineers. The architect had left the ceiling open, exposing the old-wood support beams and rafters, and he had designed the roofing out of reinforced glass. The sun quickly heated up the room, and the heat was further trapped by the insulated glass that made for a vicious cycling of the HVAC system; it was like the greenhouse effect on an office-size scale. I can only imagine what the monthly bill was to cool his office let alone the whole top floor. Bob took measures to cool it with his ceiling fan, which was of an ornate dark-wood-and-wrought-iron design. It was a good-looking fan.

He was kind enough to leave it off, knowing that most people did not like the flow of direct air blowing down on their heads as the fan was located directly above the patients' seating area. He always asked, however, once patients entered the room, whether or not they minded him turning that fan on.

No matter the weather, Bob preferred to wear a button-up sweater that he always wore unbuttoned. (Kinda like Mr. Rogers except for the buttoning part. At least he didn't wear a tie). Why anybody would wear a sweater let alone a long-sleeve shirt in that office was beyond me. He had one more odd attribute that I had not paid attention to during our first session but discovered to-day. When I came into his office this afternoon, he first asked about turning the fan on and then proceeded to ask me if I wanted a cup of hot tea. Hot tea? Really? I mean, what the fuck? It had to be eighty degrees out-side. If I wanted anything, I would've asked for a cold soft drink. As I was thinking this, he pointed over to-ward his tea machine, motioning for me to take a look.

In a cleared-out area in the corner of his office in a cleared sat a miniature white refrigerator, on top of which sat his tea machine. It looked like a brand-new commercial coffeemaker and was absolutely pristine. I mean it looked like someone had cleaned the entire unit with an electric toothbrush and toothpaste for at least a full day. Sitting around the tea machine was a small stack of miniature white napkins, a box of packets of sugar, two boxes of packets of different flavored tea, a box of plastic stirrers, and ornate ceramic teacups com-plete with cup holders. To top it off, he actually had two small, wooden chairs along the wall and next to the refrigerator. I expected to see stuffed animals on top of the chairs, but apparently someone had already taken them. The stuffed animals, that is. I was beginning to wonder who the crazy one was, not that I have a real is-sue or anything—at least not anymore. In order to avoid this whole sticky situation, I simply told him that I was not a tea drinker but thanked him anyway. I actually did like tea, but I didn't know if I'd be drinking any more anytime soon. I suddenly began to wonder if my issues were so easy to spot. Was I just an open-and-shut case of textbook depression with a hint of schizophrenia?

I offered him some advice one day right after he asked my permission to turn on his ceiling fan. I asked him why he had never tinted the glass panes that made up the roofing. He looked at me rather queerly, as if he had never heard of tinting glass before. "What exactly are you referring to, and what does it do?" Bob asked.

His question furthered my thought process about his not knowing what glass tinting was, but I went on to describe what he could do rather inexpensively. I told him that by tinting the interior windows of the roof, he could cut down on heat exposure by up to 60 percent, thus drastically reducing his cooling bills, which I imagined were quite high.

Another crease appeared in Bob's forehead as he frowned slightly while nodding his head. A double negative, I thought, but one I knew Bob was in agreement with. I noticed by the new clock on the wall that only a short time was left in our session, and we would probably go over, but Bob did not seem too concerned as he was more interested in this method of tinting the roof glass. Apparently he didn't have another appointment following mine. After explaining the details, I took it a step further and offered him the name and number of a local installer, who I was sure Bob would call shortly after I left.

"Well, I have to apologize, Mike. We've kind of gotten off track, and that's completely my fault. I greatly appreciate you talking to me about the tinting, and I can assure you that is something I will be moving forward with," he said. "I'd like to get back to the discussion involving your adoption. Is that OK?" he asked.

"Sure," I said.

"First off, you made mention that you only had one mother and also told me that you knew of no other. When you say that you knew of no other, does that meaning extend to today? I guess where I'm headed is, have you ever tried to reach out to your biological mother?" he asked.

Holy shit, where're the keys? Launch the nukes. I was so sick and freaking tired of getting asked this question that I thought I would puke. Yep, that was it. I would sit there and projectile vomit all over Bob until he was soaking wet with the fully digested double cheeseburger meal that I had for lunch. Then I'd sit and watch him puke into his trash can in utter disgust. "No," I simply replied.

"Is there a reason for that, or is it something you don't want to talk about?" Bob asked.

"No, I don't mind talking about it. It's just that, for me, anyway, my mother is my mother, and she is the only mother that I have ever known. What good would it do for me at forty-eight years of age to meet my biological mother?" I asked. "I mean, the way that I look at it, my parents fought tooth and nail to give me everything I have to date, including putting me through college—the first one in the family I might add. If I were to find out, hypothetically speaking, that my biological mother had a lot of money for some reason, I guess I would feel a bit betrayed. I guess that's it more than anything, I feel fucking betrayed by her. It's not like I have any sort of love for her. It's been forty-eight years, but one would've thought that she would have been the one to reach out to begin with, not me, not her own child who she abandoned for whatever reason."

"Well, you make a good point, Mike. I can understand what you're saying, but do you find that other people who know that you're adopted ever have a hard time, if you will, with accepting the fact that you don't know and don't plan to find out who your biological mother is?" he asked.

"Yes, you've hit the nail on the head," I said. "Anytime I have this discussion with others, mainly close friends, they're always curious about my biological mother and father and why I wouldn't want to know who they are. They usually remark something to the effect of, well, what if she has a lot of money, or what if you were to find out that you have brothers and sisters out there that you have never even met."

Bob chuckle a bit, I suppose about my comment about the money. "I'm not laughing at you, Mike. Please pardon me. I just find it interesting how rude people can be and how money seems to be such a driver in our society today," he said. "They do bring up an interesting point that I had not thought of prior to today's meeting, however, and that is the thought of you having siblings that you have never met. How does that make you feel?"

I was daydreaming again, thinking about how Bob was laughing. He's damn lucky that he said he was not laughing at me and apologized for it because had he not—let's just say that I felt like giving him a backhand across the face. "Well, that's a bit of a different story, and I'm not sure that I'm ready to go down that path just yet," I said.

"No, I completely understand, and I didn't mean to upset you in any manner," Bob replied.

"No, you're fine, you didn't upset me. Like I said, it's just not something I'm prepared to talk about right now," I responded. Bob's a pretty respectful guy. I've seen my fair share of therapists, and not too many would have apologized for a remark that really did upset me. *He is a good guy*, I thought.

"What you told me about your sister was some powerful, emotional stuff," Bob continued. "Not only in one day did you find out that you were adopted but also that your sister was adopted as well. Do you share the same feelings about your sister as you do your mother?" he asked.

"In what manner are you referring to?" I asked.

"I guess what I'm trying to understand, is where exactly you feel Debra fits into this new portrait of life that has just been painted for you," he said.

Interesting question, I thought. Again, what difference did it make if she was my biological sister or my adopted sister? Once again, I had known nothing else, and nothing had changed except that someone told me that she was adopted as well. "If I was to judge her, then I would have to judge myself; isn't that correct?" I asked.

"That's some very deep insight, and I am not the person to tell you whether you are right or wrong as I do not believe there is any right or wrong answer to this question," Bob said. "Why don't we just leave it at that for now, OK?"

"No, I've decided I want to take a step back and talk about where we left off," I said.

"That's fine, Mike. I'm sorry; what exactly are you referring to?" Bob asked.

"I want to talk about the possibility of me having a biological sibling or multiple siblings or even an extended family. When I think about adoption in those terms, it really shakes things up for me. I guess what I'm trying to say is that meeting my mother and father at this stage in my life doesn't have much meaning for me, but meeting biological siblings and relatives does for a couple of reasons I have not brought up yet," I said. "I also think it's important for you to know that I have tried to do some superficial research on who my biological parents and family may be."

"This is something that you have never admitted, at least not to me prior to now. As a matter of fact, I believe your mantra has been one of not wanting to know," Bob responded.

"I know, but in this case, I'm not sure that changing my mantra is necessarily a bad thing," I said.

"I agree. Please continue," said Bob.

"My mother has never been to see a therapist before, and she's always curious about the things that you and I discuss for an hour. She says that she doesn't understand how anyone could meet someone for the first time and start pouring out their innermost secrets, so to speak. On the way over here today, she brought the subject up again, so I decided to satisfy her curiosity. I was as open with her as I would have been with you and told her that we would probably be talking about adoption today and what that meant to me. She actually caught me completely off guard when she said that she thought it would be a good idea for me to investigate who my biological parents are and whether I have any biological siblings. I could see from the corner of my eye that she kept looking over at me while driving as if checking on what my reaction was," I said.

"What was your reaction?" Bob asked quietly.

"I felt a wave of sickness, the same sickness that I always feel when thinking about this subject matter, come over me. My palms became sweaty and so did my face along with my hairline. My heart rate increased, and I struggled to put together a cohesive sentence. I then simply came out and asked her why," I said. "My mother is a very cerebral person, and for this reason alone I was afraid of what her response would be. She told me, 'Michael, there's definitely one thing in particular that we continue to beat around the bush on, and that is the fact that I am not going to be here forever to take care of you. I know how much you hated staying at that nursing home, but unless some sort of miracle happens, that's where you're going to end up. There simply is no one else to take care of you. Maybe if you were to find out that you had some family members or relatives who actually cared, maybe they could take care of you,' she said."

"Wow, Mike. There's a lot that was both said and unsaid in her response. Do you understand what I'm talking about?" Bob asked.

"I do, but I don't know what to do or say about it. The conversation didn't go any further, as we had already been sitting out in the parking lot for a couple of minutes. I also know that once I leave here today, my discussion with her will once again take precedence as it was clear to me that it was not finalized in her mind," I said.

"Do you feel that you are currently placing a burden on her at her age?" Bob asked.

"Burden? No, I'm not placing a burden on her right now," I said. I've hired a certified nursing assistant to help me get ready in the mornings, which has taken quite a load off her. She came to me a while back and told me that she was no longer capable of doing it every day; however, she has since told me that she feels much better. My father, unfortunately, has taken a turn for the worse, and he, too, has refused to go into a nursing home, so my mother has been left to take care of him as well. Our house is like a small hospital; it can get pretty crazy at times, especially when my father does not even know where he is."

"Mike, you know what her ultimate concern is, don't you? She wants to make sure that you're taken care of after she's gone, and right now, there doesn't seem to be a plan for that, not unless you're about to tell me of one."

A wave of silence settled over our conversation. I didn't want to say what I knew had to be said next. My voice lowered to a murmur. "I have no plan." I turned to meet Bob's eyes, my voice raised, "There is no goddamn plan. When you refuse to go into a nursing home and you have no family to take care of you, your options plummet to zero rather quickly. That's really the key. After my parents pass away, I have absolutely no family that can take care of me. I'm done; game over. It's pretty much always been that way with my family though. It's always been just my mother, my father, my sister, and me—just the four of us."

"Is that what you're going to tell your mother?" Bob asked.

"Either I tell her a lie now or later—which is better? I'm not looking for an answer," I said. "Do you mind if we move on?"

"No, that's fine for now, but I'd like to talk about your father. Is that OK?" he asked.

"That's fine," I responded.

"You mentioned that, during your discussion regarding adoption with your mother, your father was not in attendance, and I noticed that you made special note of that fact," Bob said. "There seems to be something there that I don't quite understand regarding the relationship between not just you and your father but also between your sister and your father as well. I know you gave me an explanation as to why you thought he was not in attendance during that meeting, but in your mind, do you think there is a deeper explanation?"

Yeah, I knew this question was coming; it was a tennis ball lobbed straight to Bob at ten miles per hour, and he was swinging Louisville's finest large-diameter maple, ready to smash this one right out of the ballpark. I sat there for a while, pondering the best way to respond to him. "I've thought about this question time and again, and I keep coming up with the exact same answer," I said. "I honestly believe that my father viewed us as redheaded stepchildren. I can only imagine how much he must have wanted a son of his own. I don't think he was in the room that day during our discussion because he could not face rejection—rejection that may have come from either myself or my sister.

"I've never shared this with anyone besides you, but I've known it all along. I've never even told my mother, but for years now, I remember thinking what a loss it was for him to know that he had a son who loved him so deeply and only wanted the same in return. As a father myself now, I have come full circle to ponder this question on a different level. No matter how much thought I give to that question, I know that I will take it to my grave, because questioning my father for the truth may cause him great strife and bring up pain and misery that he long ago buried somewhere in his mind.

"I'm sure that if I asked people for opinions regarding why he was not with my mother on that day, I would receive a multitude of answers. I cannot say for certain that I want to know the answer to this question anyway; I can only say with certainty that I continue to ponder it. As the saying goes, 'Some things are better left unsaid.' All I know is that I will never forget that day," I said.

"I think you've made a lot of progress through the years, Mike, and I think you've reached the conclusions that best suit your situation, which is definitely a tough one," Bob said.

PANIC AT FORTY THOUSAND FEET

May 20, 1995.

My fiancée and I had not taken a vacation together in some time, mainly due to our schedules and financial situations, though some would say that living in Denver was a vacation in itself. I really can't argue this point.

My parents made the decision in the summer of 1992, the year I graduated college, to sell our home that I grew up in and move to Las Vegas of all places. My parents enjoyed gambling, but I would not say they were addicted to it by any stretch of the imagination. I do know that they loved the weather in Las Vegas relative to St. Louis. I don't know what it is about growing older, but most of the people I know that are at or near retirement have moved to warmer, drier climates. Maybe there is some truth in the idea that joints and old injuries flare up more in the wintertime than they do in the summer. I always figured it to be an old wives' tale.

While I didn't care too much for the idea of selling the home that I grew up in, there were some intrinsic benefits that we gained out of it, like being able to take a vacation without having to pay for room and board. I had already been to Vegas on several occasions, but this would be Michelle's first trip. I was the one who instigated the need for a vacation, and Michelle was amenable to the idea as long as I promised not to squander our savings on gambling, so our solution was to simply have a preset limit for each of us. Once that limit was reached (so the plan was), the gambling portion of our vacation would be over.

Just two weeks prior to us leaving, I was still ignorant of the fact that I had a chronic disease growing inside me like an alien that would slowly but surely attack and destroy my nervous system, leaving me with little in terms of functionality. I had no clue what was in store for me for the remainder of my life. This was truly a foreign disease, an opportunistic invader, an alien that I may have had since birth, but for reason unknown to even the so-called experts, this invader decided to strike me in my prime, when I was at my strongest, at the pinnacle of my life.

In March 1995, I awoke with partial vision to the blaring noise of my alarm clock. I thought for a moment that it was not morning but still nightfall. My heart raced as a searing poker-hot pain penetrated my left eye. I saw stars with each pound of my heart, pulsing and thumping blood through the arteries and veins that seemed to run deep within my eye socket behind my eyeball. I fought to grasp the alarm clock, blindly trying to find the off button because I couldn't see the words engraved on the clock. My anger and panic grew with every loud bleat from the alarm clock. I broke out in a cold, clammy sweat, grew increasingly lightheaded, and then vomited on the floor at my feet.

I sat on the side of the bed, grasping at the sheets, grasping for some explanation as to what was happening to me. My palms were sweaty and soaked the sheets clutched in my hands. I tried desperately to remain upright, but the pain was so great that I gently lay back down on the pillows. I could find no comfort; whether I sat up or lay down, the searing pain persisted.

Using my left hand, I cupped my left eye and tried to focus on the alarm clock on the nightstand. My right eye immediately focused on the red digital readout: 7:00 a.m. I realized that my right eye was not the culprit. I kept my left eye cupped and painstakingly made my way to the bathroom to choke down some pain-relief meds. In the bathroom, I sat down on the wooden toilet seat, staring down at the floor with both eyes open. My elbows resting on my thighs supported the weight of my upper body. Sweat dripped off my chest and onto my legs. In the darkness, I saw nothing but swirling colors, colors and textures mimicking the movement of the clouds in the sky. This was a very cloudy day.

My only thought at the time was that I had a brain tumor. *I must be dying*, I thought. At that moment, I wished for death as the pain was so great that not even a cocktail of acetaminophen and ibuprofen could touch it. I wanted desperately to cry, but knowing that the tears would only bring more physical pain, I sat there on the toilet seat, hunched over, staring at the linoleum floor. Worried that I was about to pass out, I knew I needed to make my way to the couch in the living room to lie down.

I had vomit on my feet, so first I needed to shower. I pulled back the plastic shower curtain and turned the water on cool. I stepped into the shower with my underpants on and lay in the tub, hunched over on my side, letting my head rest on a bath towel. I let the water fall over my body, hopefully washing off the vomit as I could barely move. Once out of the shower, I stacked up the pillows on the sectional couch to prop my head up and prevent the pounding pain.

I lay there, smelling of vomit, sweat, and fear. I was naked, cold, and soaking wet. My fear prevented me from calling anyone for help, even an ambulance. My thoughts were as murky as my vision. I closed my eyes and tried to rest. Restlessness gave way to exhaustion, and exhaustion gave way to sleep.

I awoke sometime later to the ringing of my phone. I panicked as I instantly remembered that it was a work-day, and the caller must have been my boss wondering where I was. The living room was dark; the phone continued to ring, and I lay there, afraid to open my left eye. The answering machine picked up, and I heard my boss ask where I was and kindly reminded me that not calling in to work prior to eight o'clock was a terminable offense.

Once again, I became sick, not from the tumor growing in my head but from the thought of being terminated from my first job out of college. I began to cry now, unafraid of the pain that I might feel; I wished nothing more than to be back at home, back with my mother so she could tend to me. I called no one, not even my boss. I didn't feel this tumor in my head; I felt death hanging over me.

I crawled from the couch toward the back patio door-way and lay on the cool linoleum. I knew what I needed to do but was frozen with fear. *Where is Michelle?* I wondered. *I need her. Why was this happening to me? Would Michelle leave me? Would the one person whom I loved so much walk away from me or stay by my side? Would I live long enough to find out?*

The pain that just hours before had been severe enough to cause me to vomit subsided. My only thought was that the cocktail of pain medications that I had taken had somehow done its job. Clear thought eluded me, but I knew that I must pull back the shade that covered the patio window. I knew that the final test of whether or not my vision had returned to normal lay in my ability to pull back that shade.

Hours had passed with me lying on my back before I finally built up the courage to pull back the shade and peer outside. Although still somewhat cloudy, my left eye once again recognized outlines of familiar sights that I was so glad to be able to see. I must have a vision problem, I thought. Somehow I was able to reconcile my sickness in that darkest of moments. I didn't want to go into work that day, I just wanted time; time to truly process what had happened to me, and more importantly, decide what I was going to do about it.

I finally returned my boss's phone call and proceeded to lie. I once again received the speech about termination for not calling in on time. I heard his words yet paid little attention; I had other pressing matters. Was it me, or did his voice sound muffled? I hung up the phone and contemplated this thought for some time before coming to the conclusion that I was not imagining his muffled tone. I remembered he sat next to the director of human resources and must have been concerned that his straight-*A* student had for some reason dropped the ball, dropped a bowling ball. Who gave a shit? I'd done enough. I'd proved myself worthy of my position, and I should have had nothing to be concerned about. Would he really fire me over this single incident? Why did all of this matter to me so much? After all, I had a vision problem that I needed to take care.

Several days went by with me sitting in my dimly lit apartment alone. I told my boss, Ed, that I would probably be out for the week as I was quite sick with the flu and couldn't keep my stomach in check. I could tell that, while he understood, he was upset that he would have to further explain the situation to his boss, who might not be so accepting of the situation. I envisioned his boss, Kevin, yelling at him behind closed doors to call me back to ensure that I knew that people worked all the time with the flu and that I should be treated no differently.

A slight grin came across my face as I knew that my boss did not have the balls to confront his boss directly. Most things these days were better left to e-mail correspondence. Yes, e-mail had become a way of communicating with one another while leaving all emotions out of the picture, which, of course was what we were after. While I smirked at my boss's possible plight, a deep anger, almost a rage began to overcome me. I was probably going to die, and all my boss could think of was the work that I wasn't producing, the deadlines that were not being met, and the customers that were not being satisfied.

I soon realized that I would be caught in a never-ending web of lies unless I found out what exactly was wrong with me. I could not continue with my current modus operandi and expect to keep my job; I was not being fair to either myself or my employer.

The following day, I made an emergency appointment with an ophthalmologist as I stated that I had lost vision in my left eye. I suddenly thought about the logistics of how I would get to the appointment. I could drive myself, yet that would be too risky of a situation that put other drivers at a risk they did not expect or deserve. I called my best friend and colleague at work and explained to him that I needed his help driving me to the ophthalmologist. When he asked why I wasn't able to drive myself, I told him that my vision was extremely blurry in one eye, and I did not want to risk having an accident along the way. I further pulled Mike into my web of lies and asked him for understanding when I told him that I had explained to my boss that I was sick with the flu. Why shoulder Mike with this information? I remember thinking that even he did not fully understand or believe my story; however, I knew that Mike would do whatever I asked of him.

I sat in the waiting room with Mike, again cupping each eye separately, hoping for some level of change for the better that never came. Mike sat across from me in the corner of the waiting room, reading what I believe was a *Golf Magazine*, pretending not to notice my actions, pretending not to be aware of the strange situation he had found himself in. I sat for a moment and wondered what I would do if the roles were reversed. Would I ask my best friend what the hell was going on and if he needed some help, or would I believe that I was already helping him by keeping quiet? It was obvious that Mike felt the latter, and I was glad for his help. Not too many of my other friends would have taken on such a strange request without asking a load of questions.

While sitting in the waiting room, trying to keep my mind occupied before the nurse called me, I noticed a mosaic of an old Western barn hanging from the wall. The longer I stared at the picture, the more I felt like there was something I needed to remember but couldn't. I kept having this feeling like I had been there before, not to that exact barnyard, but a feeling of familiarity with the site. It took me a few more minutes to make the connection to my first jobsite in Paris, Texas. It was there that I had my first experience with multiple sclerosis, an experience that would have otherwise fallen into the background noise of life had it not been for my current situation. The similarities between these two occasions could not be attributed to mere coincidence; there was definitely a common thread that ran through both.

The year was 1993, and I was one year out of college and already on a project site for a large client located in Paris, Texas. It was a hot, sticky summer, which made for long days inside an un-air-conditioned plant working twelve-hour shifts with fifteen- to thirty-minute breaks every four hours. We prayed for the sun to go down as we could open the plant up during the evening and get a nice, cool, strong breeze blowing through the entire building. During the days, the facility was locked up like Fort Knox, and you would've thought they were making gold there.

We were under a tight deadline and had already encountered several issues while on-site that were causing our overall project schedule to slip. We were lucky to be off the jobsite by nine or ten o'clock every evening, and that was with the scheduled start time of six o'clock sharp. When you're behind schedule and the client doesn't walk off-site, neither do you.

What had I gotten myself into? Wasn't I a white-collar engineer or at least supposed to be? Why was I working out in the field to begin with, especially under such miserable conditions? Training, I was told, was the answer—practical training that I desperately needed and that I didn't receive in college, and boy, were they right. There were no engineering classes on how to work a fifteen- to eighteen-hour shift; that just came with the territory.

I was what most of the team termed a greenhorn. That basically meant that I had no experience and everybody knew it, but it appeared that one of the goals while on-site was to prevent the client from being made aware of this fact. After all, the client was paying for top-notch experienced help, not for our company to be training me on the client's time. Either way, it really made no difference as long as the job got done at the end of every day.

Getting off work usually consisted of going back to the hotel, taking a warm shower, and climbing into bed, and, oh yeah, trying to remember to set the alarm. I remember it was a Friday evening when we were working at the plant because I know we were going to have one of our first weekends off in a long time, and that meant the team could rest up. We also knew that we were close to completion of the project, and while the work was hard, it was also rewarding to know that I would be one of the members who helped complete the project on time. I guess you could call it my first real work accomplishment.

Driving from the plant to the hotel that Friday night, four of us decided to meet up at one of the local restaurants for a good steak dinner and some beers at the bar afterward.

After dinner I went back to the hotel room, exhausted but still riding a little high, knowing that I would be returning home soon. I called my fiancée and told her the good news. I remember not having to set the alarm clock for the first time as we didn't plan to meet until lunch the next day. Around one thirty in the morning,

I awoke to a disturbing sensation in my right leg that I had never experienced before. I was not able to move it, nor was I able to feel it while touching it with my right hand. I then began to notice a completely foreign sensation of small needles being poked into my leg while it burned with waves of heat. My heart rate jumped and it pounded within my chest walls with every breath I took. What the hell was going on? Had my leg fallen asleep? If so, it had never been this bad before, plus I had never experienced the pain that came with the needle pokes. I hit my thigh with my right fist, trying desperately to get it to wake up but to no avail.

I gently made my way to the side of the bed, balancing myself on my left leg as I still had no sensation in my right leg. I had to physically pick up my right leg with my hands to ensure that my foot was touching the carpet and was firmly planted. The carpet had a completely foreign feeling as I felt every carpet fiber pricking the skin of the bottom of my foot. I continued to try to convince myself that my leg had simply fallen asleep. After about an hour of trying, I was finally able to stand upright and noticed that the feeling was beginning to return to my leg.

My leg awakening was quite painful. Each beat of my heart brought with it either the sensation of burning or being stuck with small needles. My heart rate was still rather high, and I knew that I would not be able to fall back asleep, so I decided to take a warm bath to help me relax. I fell back asleep at around four o'clock.

The following afternoon, my story made for nothing more than simple conversation over lunch. Several of the guys had other anecdotal stories, and after listening to them, I was convinced that what had happened to me was no big deal. I pushed it to the back of my mind like I had with so many other things that I didn't want to deal with.

Was what happened with my eye somehow related to what had happened to me then? The two didn't seem to be related; I mean the first occurrence had to do with my leg, and this had to do with my eyesight. No, they were just somehow strange coincidences.

"Mike? Mike Seliner?" the nurse called out for me. I raised my hand, looking over at Mike, who had a strange look about his face. I didn't know how long I had been daydreaming or how long the nurse had been calling me.

Within minutes, I was making my way to one of the rooms that lined my doctor's hallway office. Like all doctor's offices, even the ophthalmologist's had a certain smell, probably that of alcohol or other medications.

For some reason it felt different than a standard doctor's office.

I was asked to sit in one of the chairs that held a vision-testing apparatus to the left side of my armrest. I looked ahead and saw a vision chart on the wall in front of me. With my right eye, I was able to nearly see every line on the chart with my glasses on. With my left eye, I could only see patches of clearness on the eye chart. I realized that my vision had improved, but I still had a major problem.

I heard the doctor outside of my room pull my chart that sat inside a plastic file holder bolted to the wall. He spent a few minutes reading the details of my chart before knocking loudly on the heavy, solid-wood door and making his entrance. He already had a worried look about his face that caused my anxiety to climb. "Have I seen you before, Mr. Seliner?" he asked.

"No, this is the first time that I have been here," I said.

"I understand that you're having some vision problems with your left eye. Have you not been to the ER yet?" he asked.

The ER? Holy Christ, what did this man think was wrong with me? I had given them very little information when I made my appointment.

"Do you always wear glasses, Mr. Seliner?" he asked.

"Yes, I wear them for nearsightedness," I said.

"So you have not been to the ER, is that correct?"

"Correct." My world suddenly turned into a decompressing Boeing 747, and I was the only person on board. I sat in an exit row, paralyzed and unable to move; the engines were aflame. This flight was headed into an unrecoverable tailspin, and the destination lay some forty thousand feet below in a sea of darkness. Please place your seat backs in their full upright position. Close your food tray and tuck your head between your knees…ensure your seatbelts are tightly fastened and prepare for death.

Beads of sweat formed on my forehead at my hairline. I felt the sudden need for a cigarette, even though I had never smoked before. What the hell do you do on your deathbed anyway? This was no deathbed; this was a five-hundred-mile-per-hour downward spiral in a tin can with a one-way ticket straight to hell.

I heard nothing but the thumping of my heartbeat in my eardrums. My mouth instantly turned into a plantation of cotton. As my heart began to race, the blood drained quickly from my face as my body went limp; my vision began to deteriorate again.

"I'm going to shine a very bright light in your left eye first as I need to examine the optic nerve," the ophthalmologist said. A couple of eye drops washed over both my eyes. "These eye drops will cause your pupils to dilate and allow me to better see your optic nerves. I will give you a pair of clip-on sunglasses to wear for a while as any light will seem very bright and may give you a headache," he said.

Lights that seemed impossibly bright. Weren't we told not to stare at the sun in kindergarten? How could a light so bright not damage my eye?

"Mr. Seliner, I'm going to turn the room lights back on for a minute, and it may seem a little bright, OK?" he said.

The lights came on, and I noted that he was holding a black-and-white checkered placard in his right hand. The four-by-four-inch placard looked like a bingo card where the player had blotted every adjacent cell with black ink. I did not notice the magic in this trick until I was asked to cover my right eye with a large plastic spoon. My left eye focused on the center of the bingo card but saw none of its surroundings; everything else was fuzzy at best.

"Mr. Seliner, when's the last time you've been to see your neurologist?" he asked.

Neurologist? "I don't have a neurologist. What's wrong with me?" I asked.

Suddenly, the ophthalmologist stopped whatever it was he was writing and turned in his chair. He slowly rolled over to me, and I saw the paleness and emptiness in his face. "I'm sorry, Mr. Seliner. I incorrectly assumed that you were under the care of a neurologist. You have a condition in your left eye, more specifically your optic nerve, that is preventing you from seeing clearly. This condition is called optic neuritis and may last from a few days to a few months if not treated quickly."

"Am I going to lose the eyesight in my left eye? What is the treatment, and what does a neurologist have to do with it? Why can't you treat it?" I asked.

"Mr. Seliner, I don't want to panic you in any manner; however, I need to tell you that optic neuritis can be indicative of a larger disease called multiple sclerosis. I cannot say whether or not you have MS, and this is why I want you to see a neurologist. The neurologist will treat the optic neuritis with drugs called steroids, which will help shrink the swelling in the optic nerve and hopefully allow your eyesight in your left eye to return to normal. Since you have not had this condition for more than a couple days, time is on our side, but you should not wait any longer," he said.

"I don't even know a neurologist or how to find one," I said. How far were we from impact? Was there a parachute onboard? I stared at the eye chart on the wall in front of me, my left eye blind once again. The pain in my eye was on the brink of returning. I knew I was headed for tears, and so did this doctor, who most likely realized my plight also.

Apparently as an act of pity, he volunteered the names of a couple of neurologist who worked within his building and were located right down the hall. He sat on top of his little round stainless-steel chair, staring silently at me; I sat staring at the eye chart and wondering what was to become of me. Without even knowing it, the ophthalmologist had blown the lead story. He had predicted my fate. What cruel trick did this universe now have in mind for me? What of my friend Mike?

I took the business cards that I was offered and proceeded to make my way out to the receptionist where I mindlessly paid my bill.

"The doctor wants to see you in six months; is that OK?" the receptionist asked. She proceeded to search through her computer to find a date that would work for me, but the only thing I remember was saying yes. It was probably the last bill to any ophthalmologist that I would pay. I looked back across the waiting room and saw Mike still reading the magazine he had picked up when we came in. I wondered if he was actually reading it or trying to show calm in a situation that he knew was anything but.

In a single instant, I had lost everything. The plane had crash-landed, and I was the unlucky one. I was the sole survivor. I would say nothing to Mike. I would tell him that I was there for a scheduled eye exam, or had I already given him an excuse? I would tell him that my car had broken down, and I needed a ride. I knew that lie would pile upon lie, but I didn't care. At this point I would take the risk; I was willing to take any risk. Nothing mattered. I knew that Mike knew that something was wrong, but I also knew that he would not question me, and that was what I needed right then.

CHUTES AND LADDERS

Mike drove me back home from the ophthalmologist that afternoon. The doctor was right; the outdoor light was blinding. Mike engaged me in general conversation, asking me how everything went and if I was OK. Note to self: never ask a question that you are not fully prepared to hear the answer to. I really don't know if he wanted the truth or not. I don't know what he suspected. Sometimes being burdened with such an awful truth as mine can be overwhelming; it's just too much information. People matter-of-factly ask how you are doing, always expecting to hear the single-word answer, "Fine." I can't think of too many cases in which I would want to hear that someone was not doing fine but was doing horribly. Was Mike prepared to be burdened with my truth? I glanced at him as he stared mindfully at the road ahead and simply said, "Fine. Everything went as expected. I just need a new set of lenses, which are now on order."

"Good," Mike responded. "With what you described earlier, I was concerned that the issue might have been a lot worse."

Described and *issue*. These words were foreign to me, and their definition was lost in the moment. What had I told Mike about what I had experienced? Did I give him an explanation as to why I had already missed several days of work? *Think, dammit, or you may regret the words that come out of your mouth next.* Without being able to remember what I might have said to him, I remained silent for the remainder of the ride home. Mike seemed OK with that, and he too said nothing. Mike apparently had his own issues to mull over. I considered him to truly be one of my best friends, not just a colleague.

On returning to my apartment, I thanked him for his last-minute help. I closed the car door firmly and waved at him through the window, almost shoeing him away like a fly. I prayed that he would quickly drive off so that he would not notice me making a fool of myself as I trod back to my third-floor apartment; God forbid he might actually have to help me in. God was not listening to me that day however; Mike rolled the window partway down and asked if I needed any further help.

It was at that moment that I knew he suspected more, but I also knew that he would not come out and say anything directly. "No, Mike, I'll be fine. I'm sure our boss misses you more than I will," I responded with a grin on my face.

It quickly became clear that he was looking for any reason not to have to return to work. Strange, but I remember thinking that Mike was on the fast-track program toward a role in engineering management. I knew he had been working hard at climbing the corporate ladder, but he was also mindful not to let any crap fall on top of whoever was climbing the ladder behind him. No, Mike was a good friend, and he also knew that I was also being fast-tracked toward the same position. I guess one could say that we were both of equal standing, and we watched out for each other on some level, kind of like a sibling rivalry.

I wasn't sure how long of a chute this little incident would send me sliding in this game of Chutes and Ladders but hopefully not all the way back to the beginning. I would surely hate to have to give up two of my prized possessions—my Nissan 300Z and my Kawasaki Ninja 750—""proof" of my ascension on the corporate ladder.

Even in March, Denver can get quite warm, especially with no cloud cover to block the sun's rays. I don't think Denver would meet most people's expectations. When I found out that I was moving to Denver for my first job, I envisioned a city surrounded by mountains, snow, and large evergreen trees. I remember wondering why anyone would build a manufacturing facility in the middle of a ski-resort town. My ideas of this city were quickly shattered, however, as circling for landing above Denver International quickly revealed that the city was located on relatively flat land in the foothills of the Rocky Mountains. It was smack in the middle of what appeared to be a giant dust bowl.

The pollution there in the early 1990s was an absolute embarrassment to those who called Denver home, not to mention a total health hazard. I later came to learn from fellow colleagues that the dust bowl was actually composed of sand particles that were caught in an upper-atmospheric inversion of wind blowing over the mountaintops, trapping the air over Denver. During the wintertime, traditional rock salt could not be laid on the streets.—it wouldn't melt because the street surface temperatures were too low. As a result, Denver laid down sand on the roads in the wintertime, which subsequently got ground up on the pavement by car tires eventually found its way into Denver's upper atmosphere in the form of fine dust particles or pollution. Landing in the city, this collection of sand particles appeared to be the worst case of air pollution one had ever seen—worse than Mexico City if you've ever had the misfortune of flying there.

By the turn of the century, Denver had found a solution to its problem. It stopped laying sand down on the roads in lieu of a mixture of salt and a wet chemical solution that helped melt the snow and ice and also solved their larger problem of pollution once and for all.

That day's pollution level was in the red zone, and it was recommended that people remain indoors if at all possible. I had no plans to go anywhere else that day anyway. I turned down the thermostat in the apartment to a comfortable sixty-eight degrees and ensured that all the windows were shut before I sat down at my under-sized two-seater kitchen table. The table and chairs were old, remnants of the early 1970s that I pilfered from my home in St. Louis prior to moving to Denver. It was part of the deal I had worked out with my parents before my dad left for Vegas. The general plan was that he would go to move to Vegas first, and my mother would stay behind until the house sold. As luck would have it, the house sold on the day prior to my planned departure, so as a result, I had to rent my own moving truck and clear the house of whatever remained that I was allowed to take. I had already been through this process once before, back in college, so there really wasn't much of anything left after my parents took what they wanted.

So at the age of twenty-four, I loaded up the U-Haul with all my belongings and proceeded to make the trek out to Denver, some nine hundred miles away. I clearly recall no one being home, not even my friends, on the day that I left for Denver. I took one look back, standing out in the middle of our street, looking at the neighborhood and remembering my friends who had played such an integral role in defining me. I wondered if I would ever be back.

Now, back in my apartment in Denver, I reached up and grabbed the telephone off the kitchen countertop and set it directly in front of me on the table. My apartment itself was naturally dim as the only sunlight that penetrated the living room and made its way back to the kitchen came from the back sliding-glass door. I had a five-foot by five-foot wooden deck that was cantilevered off the back side of the building, and while it wasn't legal, I grilled my fair share of steaks on my hibachi. I grabbed the two neurologists' business cards that the ophthalmologist had given to me and slowly looked them over. Each doctor simply held the title neurologist, and each practiced out of the same suite.

The last time that I had been to a doctor was for a simple ear infection at the age of around ten, and that doctor was my PCP. To say that I was a typical male regarding my usage of doctors was an understatement. I had probably been to see the dentist more than I had seen any doctors. I had been a healthy young man.

After contemplating which doctor to call, I picked up the receiver, started dialing, and then quickly hung up, realizing I had no idea what I wanted to say. It was pretty plain and simple—all I wanted to do was make an appointment. It was the receptionist that I was calling, not the neurologist directly. My palms were sweaty, and my heart rate had increased, both for good reason.

I grabbed the receiver once again and dialed one of the neurologists. I spoke with the receptionist, who quickly transferred me to the doctor's nurse with whom I held a lengthy conversation. I did most of the talking. I explained that the ophthalmologist had given me good reason to believe that I had multiple sclerosis and that I was experiencing what he had termed an "exacerbation." Christ, I thought, I didn't even know the meaning of the word exacerbation. I didn't even know what MS really was.

After some back-and-forth regarding how and why the ophthalmologist had come to this conclusion, the nurse set an appointment for me to meet with the neurologist the following week. She further indicated that if I was in the middle of an exacerbation, it was important that they begin treatment as early as possible in order to prevent any possible damage to my optic nerve. I understood what she said; it all made sense, but what did treatment involve?

I realized after hanging up the receiver that my goal of climbing the corporate ladder and becoming an engineering manager at my young age was foolish; it was the least of my concerns now. My thoughts spun out of control as I wondered how I would get back home; that was where I wanted to be. My God, I thought, where is home now? I no longer had a home as I had remembered it some years ago. Where would I find that comfort that I so desperately yearned for at the moment? My parents, who had since moved to Las Vegas, could not in any way find out about this.

My web of lies was exponentially increasing in size. People, friends, my family were already being snared in my web of lies, unbeknown to them. I felt nothing. I was alone at a moment in time in which I desperately needed to be surrounded by those who loved me, yet all I could think about was how to prevent them from finding out my secret.

SUPERMAN

Superman was a childhood hero of mine. Not to the extent that I collected action figures or memorabilia of any sort, but he was just a general hero I admired. Hearing that on June 1, 1995, Christopher Reeve had been injured in a horse-riding tournament turned my world upside down. For hours that turned into days, the press was kept out of the loop as to the extent of his injuries. The only news on the Internet was silent video clips of the riding accident. To watch the tragedy unfold in slow motion made me clench my jaws and grind my teeth in despair. Fellow riders and news commentators alike painted a gruesome and heartbreaking picture that made one wonder whether he was actually still alive.

When the story finally broke, and it was clear that Superman had instantly become a quadriplegic on a respirator, it undermined the rules of the universe for me. Again, that nagging question…how could God let a tragedy like this unfold? I blamed the only person I could. Christopher was not just injured; he could not even breathe on his own without the help of a respirator. This story pierced my heart like a silver bullet, and I knew exactly why. It was the clash of the Titans, good versus evil, and this time, evil had won. Evil had won in such an overwhelming and brazen manner; this was no simple loss.

A hero is an ordinary individual who finds the strength to persevere and endure in spite of overwhelming obstacles.

— Christopher Reeve

I once again saw nothing. Like the blindness that had struck me down so hard just a short time ago, I was left partly senseless. I know what blindness had done and continued to do to my psyche, and I was left wondering what Christopher was feeling. I was left wondering what his family was thinking. Here was a man, a superhero, who could no longer lift even his own finger.

Superman was no stranger to loss in his comics and movies, but what was the man behind the mask thinking now? Was he left to wallow in his own self-pity like me, or was he prepared to fight? In my mind, I envisioned only one outcome for Mr. Reeve and his family—he would fight. This paralysis was his real-life kryptonite, and somehow he would figure out a way to break free.

When Christopher finally made his first public appearance after the riding accident, I could not help but see the parallels in the manner in which he was rolled out on stage in front of an eagerly awaiting audience and the manner in which Hannibal Lecter was bound in a straitjacket, strapped to a cargo dolly, and rolled out onto the Memphis International Airport tarmac in the movie *The Silence of the Lambs.*

Christopher was motionless. He was lifeless. He was immobile. Why? How could this happen? I was unable to take my eyes off the spectacle that was unfolding in front of me on the television. His wife by his side, he sat stoically upright in his wheelchair and spoke quietly into the microphone that was just millimeters from his lips. His wife gently held his hand, and her love for him was obvious. A deafening silence fell over the crowd as they awaited his first words. He took in a large breath of air, chest expanding, and began to speak. His speech, while short, focused on the good that lay ahead for him and his family. He fully recognized the fact that the road would be long and difficult; however, he also acknowledged the lesser-known fact that research on spinal cord injuries was helping to make progress in healing the injured every day. He was determined, not just with words but with what seemed to be an inner strength that I cannot clearly define, that he would one day move again, starting with his index finger.

Incredible, I thought. This hero to me, to so many others, had just stared death in the face, and he was already planning his recovery! Like so many that day, I cried. I wept privately, behind closed doors. I cried for my hero—or was I taking pity on myself for what I thought one day lay ahead for me as well? I felt a knot in my throat. Anger built inside me. This anger quickly turned to rage, and that proverbial knot in my throat prevented me from swallowing. I began to choke on a rage that grew from pity, not for the man and his family, but for me. But did either of us deserve this misdirected pity?

March 30, 2007.

"Can you tell me, Mike, how strong your faith is?" Bob asked.

"Do you mean in God?" I asked.

"Yes," Bob said.

"That's a good question, and I'm not sure that even at this stage in my life I can give you a good, honest answer," I replied.

"I know that you were raised in a Catholic family, and it sounds like your faith had a strong impact on your life at least through grade school from what you've told me. I'm just trying to understand if you feel that your faith has dropped off in any manner during your life, especially as it pertains to your disease," Bob said.

"Yeah, I understand exactly what you're talking about, and I guess the more that I think about it, I would tell you that the best answer I could give you is that I believe in a higher being, call Him God if you wish. After grade school and into high school and even college, I would say that I did not lose my faith; however, I simply didn't practice it. I mean I never attended church during those times, and while my father and mother still prayed to God prior to every meal we ate, that was about the extent of it. Does that make sense to you?"

"Yes, it does. I know that our faith can wax and wane during times of, call it turmoil, or where we may have a change of life in general, such as going off to college and losing daily touch with your family and your church," he replied.

"To be honest, when I was first diagnosed, I struck out at my God in anger. Not that I was a practicing Catholic to begin with, but I was looking for something, someone to lash out at. Unfortunately, that someone was my God. I can tell you that I've since come full circle to once again praise Him. There is no longer a moment that goes by in my life in which I don't try to understand how all the pieces of this cosmic puzzle fit together," I said. "I'm happier now, and He brings peace to my heart."

Then Jesus declared, "I am the bread
of life. Whoever comes to me will
never go hungry and whoever believes
in me will never go thirsty."

— (John 6:35)

I told Bob that I had gone to see a new psychiatrist a few days before, and like everything else, he asked why I had done so.

"As you're aware, I had to recently change my insurance provider mainly due to me going on disability," I said. "If it hadn't been for that, I probably still would have been with Dr. Greciah."

He responded by asking me how I liked my new psychiatrist and how my first appointment went. I told him that I kind of liked him because he seemed to have a sense of humor, which I had not found in other psychiatrists.

"How is that, Mike? How did he have a sense of humor that you found appealing?" he asked.

"Well, first off, his demeanor was relaxed, which helped put me at ease. I didn't want to be there at all, and I think he noticed. I'm sure he gets this from a lot of his patients or, I should say, that psychiatrists in general usually do," I said. "For the first time ever, and I do mean ever, he didn't bother to ask me what medications I was currently taking."

"Why do you bother to make a point of this?" Bob asked.

"Because every time I have a new appointment with a new doctor, I always print out a full list of the current medications that I'm taking," I said. A thin veil of embarrassment rushed over me, and I must have blushed because I realized that I had given Bob this very list when I first met him. He too had fallen victim to asking the same question, and I had supplied him with a complete list. Kinda makes you wonder if anyone is really paying attention. I didn't say anything further about it as I didn't want to embarrass either of us any more than I already had. That was not my intent, so I just let the subject lie. Bob could interpret it or try to remember whether he had asked me that question on his own time.

Bob, however, was quick to point out the fact that he had asked me what medications I was already on right after I had given him the list. He said, "You probably think I'm an idiot like all the rest, don't you?" Then he laughed out loud. "Sorry, just joking out loud, Mike. Don't take it the wrong way, please."

I began to laugh too. "No harm, no foul, Bob, but you have to admit it's funny nonetheless," I said. "Anyway, after going through my antidepressive-medication collection, he asked how Abilify had been working for me. I told him that I thought that while it provided some help, it didn't do anything spectacular for me. He started laughing out loud while covering his mouth, and the whole situation left me kind of confused as to what was so funny. Dr. Billes apologized and said that the whole issue with Abilify was, quite honestly, a complete joke. I was about to be exposed to some psychiatric humor, and boy, was it dry.

He said that if I had paid any attention I would have seen advertisements for that very drug out in the waiting room. He asked me if I was aware of the overpopulation of advertisements that were in magazines, billboards, and on the air. I told him that I had noticed and thought that I had read somewhere that Abilify was initially given as a sleep aid. I asked him if that was true. "How do you go from sleep aid to antidepressant?" I asked him.

Dr. Billes responded that I was right; it was initially dispensed as a sleep aid, but immediately after that, it was dispensed as an antischizophrenic medication. Now that truly is crazy. There's an advertisement for Abilify sitting out in the waiting room, and out of all people, who do they have as their spokesperson? Abraham Lincoln!

"The insanity of the whole situation just made me laugh," I said to Bob. "Dr. Billes went on to further state that the FDA and the pharmacologist from the drug company had found more use in the drug as a bump to basically any antidepressant. But what really made me laugh was the fact that Abraham Lincoln was advertising the drug. I didn't read the whole advertisement, but it was probably something about how well the drug

works, and that's no lie! Other than that, his entire office and waiting room was nothing short of a madhouse,
and the decorum needed some help as well."

"What do you mean? What was so different about
the two offices?" Bob asked.

"Well, for starters, the waiting room had to be
about ten times larger than your office alone, which
is no small room," I said. "Secondly, there was a train
of people coming in and out of the offices, and I say
offices because it appeared that there were at least a
half-dozen doctors working that day. And third, this
waiting room wasn't like any other waiting room I
had been in before. The entire room was wall-to-wall
white linoleum tiling with painted white walls and a
white drop-down ceiling with bright florescent lights.
I would have had no problem with anyone wearing
sunglasses inside that waiting room or being in a straitjacket. I was surprised to see that the walls weren't
padded with white insulation. There was enough conversation occurring between the waiting patients that
you would have thought that a group-therapy session
was taking place. On entering the room, I honestly
thought I was in the wrong room, and I was a bit
embarrassed as everyone stopped momentarily and
turned to look at me. They quickly went back about

their business, and it wasn't until then that I realized that it was just a bunch of patients talking among themselves. Anyway, it was funny stuff that I thought you'd get a kick out of."

Bob responded by literally laughing out loud at the scene I had described and how something like that would never be satisfactory to him or his colleagues.

"I'd like to talk a minute about your meeting with the ophthalmologist if you don't mind, OK?" he asked.

"Sure. What else would you like to know?" I asked.

"I'd like to talk about your friend—I believe his name was Mike also?" Bob asked.

"Yeah, his name was Mike. He was a good friend and colleague from work. I actually went to the University of Missouri, Rolla, with him but didn't really know him then. I should say that I really never met him there," I said.

Bob said, "You mentioned that you guys were friends and colleagues, so I'm interested in knowing why you made the conscious decision to not tell him what was going on with you at the time. Were you worried that he would betray you in some manner or tell others about your disease? He seemed like your one way out of a sticky situation."

I stared past him out the window to the right of his desk at an old man loading boxes into one of those pay-by-month storage garages. I was daydreaming again, ignoring the question that had been asked. I guess I had no reason and therefore, no answer. I was wondering what that man had in all those boxes that were so important that he felt he had to store them. Why was he storing versus selling whatever was in them?

I remember watching a reality television program on cable that I believe was called *Storage Wars*. It was about teams of people who traveled to sites where auctions were held for storage garages on which people had defaulted on their monthly payments and apparently could no longer be contacted to be advised that their personal belongings were about to be auctioned off. I recall seeing some garages filled with absolute garbage while others were filled with pristine personal belongings. What happened to these people? Did they die perhaps? Or maybe they just moved on in life—went through a divorce and never looked back?

"There's something that you should know about me, Bob, in case you haven't already drawn the conclusion. I'm a pretty solitary person. I don't auction off the contents of my life to the lowest bidder. I know it may sound strange, but it's just who I am," I said. "Mike was a friend of mine, that's true, but I guess I still viewed him as work competition. He and I were vying for the same position at work, and we both reported to the same boss, and I guess somehow I felt that being diagnosed with this disease would immediately disqualify me from the opportunity that lay ahead. I was a competitor with a type-A personality. I still am a competitor; I don't like to lose," I said.

"It's sad to me now when I reflect back on it," I continued. "As a matter of fact, I can honestly say that it disgusts me to think about my behavior toward my own friend. Do you know that after I told him about my diagnosis, he did absolutely nothing but try to help in every way possible? I feel horrible for thinking that he would somehow cheat me out of something that I had worked so hard to obtain. Instead he did the opposite. He took time out of his own life to help me in my time of need to stay afloat. I'm proud to say, however, that my ways have changed, at least when it comes to having an open conversation about my disease. For this, I have no one to thank but Mike."

"That's great to hear, and I know firsthand how much strength it takes to create open and honest change like you went through," Bob said. "How about your wife? Where was she at the time?"

"Well, my fiancée was still living in St. Louis at the time. She only visited me during the summertime and as time permitted during her studies. At my urging, and for her financial benefit, she decided to obtain her masters in social work. I convinced her that there really was no money to be made in social work without a master's degree. Going through an incident like the one that I did, well, let's just say it wasn't tailor-suited for a long-distance phone conversation or explanation," I said. "It wasn't like I planned to keep this a secret from my fiancée; I was just waiting for the proper timing, thus the vacation to Las Vegas."

Bob replied with a standard psychology-101 answer. "You know how important it is to not keep things bottled up inside, don't you, Mike?"

"Of course I do, and looking back on it now, I realize what I was doing to myself and how destructive my own behavior was to my psyche. I don't know why for sure, but I need help, help in not only understanding why I have a complete lack of trust in people, but also why I refused to tell anyone about my disease," I said. "For Christ's sake, I didn't even have a plan for telling my employers what was going on with me let alone what to do for the rest of my life should I be diagnosed with multiple sclerosis."

CHOICES AND CONSEQUENCES

May 23, 1995.

My fiancée and I left my parents' condo and headed to Treasure Island, off the main strip in Las Vegas for some R and R shortly after lunch. I needed to be alone with my thoughts, so I headed to the blackjack tables, one of my favorite games. Michelle wanted to go shopping, so we agreed to meet back up at the entrance at around three thirty.

I once again began to see this tragedy unfold in black and white. The colors that had made life so pleasant for a brief moment began to vanish. My analytical mind had taken over for the time being. It was safer that way; no one would get hurt, and answers to complex questions lay in the simplest of binary code. Throughout my life, I had come to see many things as a flip of a coin, a power switch on a computer, yes or no, on or off, true or false. My life had revolved around an elementary statistic—fifty-fifty. I had reasoned that the odds were at least 50 percent that I would be diagnosed with multiple sclerosis. "The odds of Mike Seliner being positively diagnosed with multiple sclerosis are equal to or greater than fifty percent."

The equation was flawed, however, as I had already been diagnosed with optic neuritis. I needed to add a variable to my equation, but I didn't know what the odds were on having optic neuritis. How did having optic neuritis affect the odds of having MS? My future lay in the statistical game of coin toss; I didn't care for the odds too much.

I began to daydream about the test I had done in Denver prior to us coming to Las Vegas. The radiologist offered me a shot of something to help me relax, some sort of benzodiazepine I'm sure, probably Valium. I wasn't a big fan of drugs, not even aspirin, which is certainly ironic based on my intake of drugs today.

"The scan is probably going to last about one hour in total, Mr. Seliner. Do you think you'll be OK with that, or do you think you'll need to come out of the MRI for a short break?" the radiologist asked.

"I think I'll be fine," I responded in my most manly posture possible.

"We'll give you a pair of earplugs as it will get very noisy inside the MRI, but that's normal, nothing to be concerned about. We will also be blowing in fresh oxygen from the top opening of the MRI over your head, and that should also help to relax you. If you start to feel sick or get claustrophobic, all you have to do is let us know. There is a built-in microphone inside the MRI near your head, and we will be able to take immediate action," she said.

Jesus, I thought, the test sounds worse than the disease. "How long will it take to get the results from the test, and what exactly are you looking for?" I asked. I recalled what the doctor had told me prior, but I wanted to make sure that the radiologist was telling me the same thing. If anything, I've always been somewhat paranoid. Each of us has some sort of problem, some glitch in the matrix.

"Well, the MRI will give us the imaging immediately on completion, however the supervising radiologist will need to interpret the results, write them up, and then send them off to your neurologist," she said. "Usually the whole process only takes about three to five days."

Only takes about three to five days? I felt my life was hanging on the line, and she made it sound like that was such a short period of time. No, she used the wrong adjective—three to five days was a lifetime. Three to five days of waiting, thinking, and mulling over the possibilities of what my future might hold for me. How can anyone be a radiologist? Going on vacation would interrupt my train of thought. I was glad to be leaving shortly after the tests.

MRI. I've heard the acronym used several times now to describe a machine that performs tests to look for so-called plaque or lesions on my brain and cervical spinal column that can be indicative of MS. I had done my homework beforehand but had never had an MRI before. The acronym MRI stands for magnetic resonance imaging. It is a noninvasive medical test that physicians use to diagnose a wide variety of medical ailments. MRI uses a powerful magnetic field, radio-frequency pulses, and a computer to produce detailed 3-D pictures of organs, soft tissues, bone, and virtually all other internal body structures. In many cases, MRI gives different information about structures in the body than can be seen with an x-ray, ultrasound, or computed tomography (CT) scan.

For an MRI test, the area of the body being studied is placed inside a special machine that contains a strong magnet. (What they fail to tell you is that not just the area of the body being studied but the entire body is placed inside the machine). In some cases, contrast material may be injected into the bloodstream during the

MRI scan to show certain structures more clearly. For an MRI scan exploring lesions both on the brain and cervical spine, contrast material is almost always used.

After the radiologist explained how the procedure itself would work, she walked me over to a men's dressing room where I was asked to remove my clothing and place on a gown. Apparently this was done to ensure that I had no ferrous metal (metal with iron in it) on me, as the magnets used in the MRI are so strong that they can actually pull ferrous metal out of your body during the procedure, which can be life-threatening. Not to worry though, as almost all metal that is placed within the body is nonferrous in nature and is usually made from titanium because of its lightweight strength properties. I must've been asked whether or not I had any metal in my body and what exactly the procedure was no less than five times. I was then escorted down the hallway by the nurse to the MRI room where a lighted sign above the door read, "Magnet in Use." Next to that was a small, cylindrical red light surrounded by a metal cage that also lit up when the magnet was in use.

Behind the large, solid-wooden double doors and inside the room that housed the MRI machine, I saw the lead-lined window with the row of computer monitors and technicians staring back at me, waiting to get the whole process started. The lead-lined glass had an odd green tint to it, making it appear as though we were under water. Was this just another routine day for them? Another patient among the hundreds, perhaps thousands, that each of them imaged this year alone? Did they have any empathy for their patients as they watched the results come to life on their monitors? Or did they talk among themselves about what they were having for dinner that night?

The nurse asked me to lie down headfirst on the table that would feed me into the MRI machine. The nurse asked me if I would like a blanket as it was rather cool inside the room, which I declined; I knew the contrast material would make me sweat. She gave me a set of earplugs that I promptly placed into my ears before they swung a plastic cage over my face that was just about an inch or so away from my nose. The cage reminded me of a door on a bird's cage except that it was plastic.

The nurse pressed a couple of buttons on the side of the MRI machine, and the table slowly fed me into the unit where I elevator tunes played and oxygen blew rapidly over my face from the top of my head. Now I understood why they were asking if I was claustrophobic! The MRI machine reminded me of nothing short of a Pratt & Whitney gas-turbine airplane engine (at least the housing).

I then heard the crackle of a microphone speaker come on, and the nurse asking if I was OK. After a couple of assurances to her that I was fine, she told me that there would be several tests performed, and that the first one would last approximately fifteen minutes. She told me that while the test was running, I would hear a loud series of noises and that they were perfectly normal, and I should not be concerned about them. She also indicated that it was of the utmost importance that I remain perfectly still, or they would have to redo the tests. This point was not lost on me as I had no intention of repeating this test.

The noises that the machine made could have easily matched those of a Pratt & Whitney engine less earplugs—of that I am positive. I'm sure that the radiologists were watching my brain and spine pop up in full 3-D resolution on their monitors, and perhaps they were talking among themselves about it. "Jesus, look at this poor bastard. He's screwed for the rest of his life, and he doesn't even know it yet."

I tried to think of a peaceful place in my mind and focus as I knew it would take an hour, and we hadn't even passed fifteen minutes yet. This was the first time in my life that I felt I was not in control of my situation or surroundings. I tried to convince myself that I was fine, but in reality, I was not. I could only imagine how a claustrophobic person would handle being in such tight quarters as this machine. There is simply no way; there has to be an alternate method. Maybe that's why they asked me if I wanted the drugs. Maybe they're used to people freaking out inside this cold plastic tube. Did I make a mistake by not asking for the drugs?

As the MRI ran through its normal diagnostic procedures, it created different deafening sounds with each start-stop cycle. The noises were akin to Dr. Seuss describing the possible noises that a broken synthesizer might make. Being an engineer, I could not help but wonder who invented the machine and how they did it. I had once heard that the machine was invented during the space race to the moon. Fact or fiction, I'll never know. Who was the test monkey? An actual monkey? But monkeys don't lie still unless they're drugged out. I remember that being the only laugh that I had during the experience—a picture in my head of a whacked-out monkey lying inside that tube, not knowing what the hell was going on but also not giving a flying shit—the drugs were good that day.

We came home from Treasure Island that afternoon and I headed straight up to the spare bedroom to take a nap prior to going back out for dinner. Only those living with MS can appreciate the body and mind's constant need for sleep and energy replenishment. For me, anyway, it has always been nearly impossible to go more than ten straight hours without a substantial nap. Another side effect that often brings the body to a crawl is heat. Even temperatures within the eighties and especially direct sunlight can drain the life force right out of you.

I closed the bedroom door behind me, got undressed, and slipped under the cool bedsheets, letting my head fall back onto the plush goose-down pillow. The window curtains were open, but little light was coming in as a severe thunderstorm was quickly making its way toward the house.

From where my parents lived, I could see the commercial airplanes stacked up and neatly spaced, one behind the other, waiting for landing clearance into McCarran International Airport. It was only in that moment that I truly realized and appreciated how mechanical and automated the entire process of directing air traffic around the airport was. It was a perfect symphony of air-traffic controllers all doing their jobs in perfect harmony. As I stared at the landing lights off in the distance, the rain began to come down in sheets, obscuring the view of the planes. Almost immediately, the smell of fresh rain made its way into the bedroom, and the blowing air conditioner muffled the voices of my parents in the kitchen below. Within minutes I was sound asleep.

I awoke several hours later to my fiancée's gentle voice whispering in my ear that it was time to get up, that it was time for dinner. I opened my eyes and stared at her as she sat over me looking back, waiting for me to fully awake. I knew her eyes were hazel, but I had never noticed the minute areas of slightly mixed colors that made her eyes all the more beautiful. At that moment, I was overcome by a sensation of deep love and need to be with her in a manner that I had never been before. I grabbed her as she sat on the edge of the bed and gently lifted her over me and lay her down on the bed directly next to me. I buried my face into the back of her long, ruffled hair and tried to fight back the tears that welled up in my eyes and dripped into her hair. She had such thick hair, and I couldn't prevent myself from running my fingers through her hair whenever I had the chance. Now was one of those times that I just wanted to bury my face in her hair and smell the sweet perfume on her neck. Her perfume permeated her hair, and it relaxed me.

She hated having her hair messed up, me removing her scrunchies. She always squirmed around and tried to face me, to kiss me, but this time I held back and simply buried my face in the pillow behind her neck, holding her tightly to my chest. I know she sensed something was wrong as she felt me struggle to maintain a normal breathing pattern. I was fighting back the tears, fighting back the emotional outburst that I knew I was on the brink of. She quickly turned around within my grasp, stared at me with her mouth hanging slightly open, and gently asked me what was wrong.

I slowly turned away from the pillow, stared into her eyes, and said, "I think I am really sick."

"What do you mean? Are you sick to your stomach?"

I thought for a moment about how easy a cure for an upset stomach would be. I couldn't help but laugh. It was not the laughter of joy; it was laughter at the absurdity of what she was thinking versus what I was about to tell her. I tried to regain my composure as I didn't want anyone outside the room to hear the sentence that I was about to deliver. "No, Michelle, I wish it was as simple as a stomachache. I've been sick for some time now but didn't realize the severity of my situation. I purposely chose to ignore the silent symptoms that were coming and going for about the past two years."

Michelle simply lay there, her grasp drawing tighter around me, intently focused on the words that I was nervously uttering. A pause in my confession prompted her to ask me to please continue, that she was listening, and that whatever it was, we would fight it together.

My pause gave way to reflection as I stared past her at the raindrops that were collecting on the bedroom window. A sudden flash of worry came over me. I knew in that exact moment that what I was about to say would either make her stay and fight with me—fight a disease that neither of us knew anything about—or simply walk away. What would I do? The answer was so simple for me. I loved this woman I was about to marry, and no matter what, I would fight for her; I would be there for her. Could the same be said of her?

"Michelle, last week before we came down here for vacation, I had an MRI done. Have you ever heard of an MRI? Do you know what it's for?"

"Yes, I have heard of it. Tell me why you had one done. Please tell me what's happening."

"I had it done because my neurologist believes that I may have multiple sclerosis. Do you know what MS is?"

She said nothing. Her bottom lip quivered as it always did prior to her beginning to cry. The tears welled up in her eyes, and she put her cheek to mine and began to gently cry. She whispered in my ear the words that I had been waiting for days to hear. "I am so sorry, Michael. Please know how much I love you and that I would never leave you. We will fight this disease together."

She backed away from me, holding my face in her hands, crying and staring into my eyes. She continued to speak, and I watched her lips move, but I couldn't force myself to listen any longer; I was physically and emotionally drained. She had already spoken the words that provided me with so much comfort, and I knew that I would not be left alone. Once again, I pressed my chest to her back and fell asleep in her loving arms. Dinner would have to wait.

Silence Isn't Always Golden

I awoke several hours later to my fiancée still lying next to me, holding my hands, wide awake. Her face came into focus as she gently whispered, "It's time to wake up, Michael." The sickness of worry washed over me again. For a few peaceful hours, I had dreamed of nothing, but now I was back to reality. The sandman had come and gone and left me with nothing but reality to deal with. It wasn't fair.

The doctor had told me that it would take a few days to get my test results back, and I had already been on vacation for a week. We had made prior plans to go to the Mirage for a nice dinner and a show featuring Siegfried and Roy. I was looking forward to seeing the show as every other time I had been to Vegas, I did nothing but gamble. Jesus, what if someone from work had been trying to get ahold of me this past week? I decided to check my voice mail prior to walking out the door.

I quickly made my way through the minutia of voice mails when I was stopped in my tracks by one from my neurologist. "Hello, Mr. Seliner, this is Dr. Hammond." I had been holding my breath, and a great wave of heat came over my body as my forehead began to sweat at the hairline. It suddenly felt like it was eighty degrees Fahrenheit inside our condominium. Fifty-fifty, I thought to myself. "I'm calling to let you know that your test results were positive. We did find a lesion on the brain and one in your cervical spine. As soon as you are able, please call my office and set up an appointment so we can discuss a plan for moving forward," he said.

Suddenly that heat wave turned to cold, and I began to shiver. The beer that I had been holding by the neck slipped out and smashed onto the kitchen flooring. My parents were in the room with me sitting at the kitchen table, waiting for me to hang up the phone so we could go out. My back was toward them, and I leaned over the counter to help support my weight as my knees began to buckle. When did I give my work number to Dr. Hammond, or did I? I repeated the message for a second time, listening for that key word *positive. My life is over…My life is over*; the words ran on a loop in my mind that I couldn't stop.

"My God, Michael, are you OK?" my mother shouted.

I hadn't noticed that I was standing in a puddle of beer and broken glass, the neck label still pinched between my index finger and thumb. The pressure on my eardrums was immense, and I was having trouble hearing my mother speak to me. All signs of going into shock; all systems go; let go, Michael.

"Michael, are you OK?" she asked again.

My breathing was shallow, yet my heartbeat was hard. All six foot two inches of my mainframe wanted to go crashing to the floor.

"Yes, yes, I'm all right. The label on the top of the beer bottle just slipped off from being wet. I'll clean it up; don't worry," I responded with my back still toward her. I hung the phone up and went over to the sink to get a wet washcloth and to the pantry for a broom and dustpan.

Michelle met my glance back at the kitchen table met. She hadn't said a word. She knew what had occurred; she knew the unfortunate truth. I stared back down at the mess on the floor and began to clean it before my mother came over and finished the job. It was just like her to clean up someone else's mess. I sat down at the kitchen table and pulled my boots off prior to heading upstairs.

"Where are you going?" asked my father. "We need to get moving if we plan on making dinner and the show on time."

The spider web was about to double in size and the lies triple in complexity. "I'm just running upstairs to get cleaned up. I need a clean pair of pants. I'll be back down in a few minutes."

Michelle followed me up to the bedroom. I walked in the room; shut the door behind her; and sat at the foot of the bed, staring at the floor.

The world isn't all sunshine and rainbows. It's a very mean and nasty place, and I don't care how tough you are, it will beat you to your knees and keep you there permanently if you let it. You, me, or nobody is gonna hit as hard as life. But it isn't about how hard you hit, it's about how hard you can get hit and keep moving forward.

— Rocky Balboa

"Are you telling me that your doctor left you a voice mail regarding your medical results?" Michelle asked. "What did he say? Did you save it on your voice mail? Please, Michael, don't stop talking to me now. Please stay with me. I need you now. I need you as much as you need me. I told you we would get through this together," she said.

"It's over," I said. "Yes, he did leave a voice-mail message for me, and yes, they did find lesions on my brain and cervical spine. He wants me to make an appointment with him as soon as I get back so that we can discuss plans going forward."

She hugged me tightly, pressing her cheek up against mine, "Michael, I am so sorry. I love you so much, and you know that I will never leave you," she said.

That night would be our last night in Vegas. Again I lied and told my parents that work needed me back for issues with a project that I had been working on. My parents had already grown to understand that, for me, work came above all else—how unfortunate. This spider had just woven a few more intricate designs in its web of lies.

My parents dropped us off at the airport after a dinner where virtually no words were spoken, at least none that I can remember; I had too much on my mind. I did, however, apologize emphatically about having to leave early, which my father seemed to understand more than my mother. I believe he understood because I was more like him than I wanted to admit. Prior to his retirement, his work was his life. Again, how unfortunate. So much time wasted dealing with so many issues that made no difference in the end.

Once we arrived at the boarding gate, we had an approximately hour-and-a-half wait as we were trying to board an earlier flight than our scheduled one. All of the seats at the gate were empty except for a few people who were either waiting for friends and family to show or waiting to board the same flight back to Denver as we were. Michelle and I sat in front of the large ceiling-to-floor windows that overlooked the gate and runway as we both had some nostalgia for planes.

Perhaps it was because I had given her a promise ring at a beautiful restaurant that sat next to the east end of the runway in St. Louis. I sat outside by the large fire pit, watching planes come in for landing while holding her hand. We were young and deeply in love; time seemed irrelative. It was a special night that she in no way expected, and one that I didn't expect to pull off so well. That was the true beginning of our relationship, and I'm sure we were both thinking of that moment now, at the Las Vegas airport. I never asked; I just sat slumped down in the chair, staring out at the planes that were taking off.

Nighttime was falling, and so was a misty rain. I reached up to grab Michelle's hand and met hers partway. We had so much in common. I truly believed that we knew what the other was thinking.

Once back in Denver, I knew that there was only one place that I needed to be. I had to fulfill my curiosity for knowledge, to know all there was to know about multiple sclerosis. I had not been to the library since my early years in college. For me, the library was not just a place to study but a hideout of sorts, a fortress of solitude. I would have to wait until the next day, however, as it was close to midnight by the time we finally got home and settled in.

The following day, I drove from our apartment to the nearest library that I could remember. At the time, GPS units were meant for the military and maybe the super-rich—certainly not me. I recalled an older several-story high public library being located behind the grounds of a recently built strip mall. As the building came into sight, I was happy to see that it had not succumbed to the wishes of the strip-mall developers.

It was early morning when I pulled into the back of the parking lot and turned off my ignition. I sat, absorbing the complete silence that I so desperately needed. I had not slept well the night before.

I laid my head back on the headrest, reclined the seat back to a comfortable position, and put in my favorite CD. I listened to the music with my eyes closed and my windows partway down. I thought about what lay ahead; I could go or stay, the decision was completely up to me. I could wait to get the answers to my questions at my doctor's follow-up visit.

I had no idea how long the library was open on a Saturday as I had not been in so long. I tried to remember what it was like inside besides all of the books. Who did I need to meet to help me gather the information I was looking for? I didn't even own a library card; how could I even get in? As my brain went into overdrive, I could find no rest and decided it would be best to head inside.

I wondered for a brief moment whether the librarian was aware of my fate when I asked her for all the material they had on multiple sclerosis. I would say that the look on her face was one of shock and concern, not for me, but for the amount of work it would apparently take to pull together all of the material I had requested. I walked with her down three winding flights of open staircases located in the center of the cylindrical building. From the vantage point of the staircase, I could see around each level of the library.

The silence in the building was broken by the click-clacking of her high heels on the slick marble slabs of the staircase. Her perfume was overwhelming, probably masking a bad smoking habit, I thought.

We came up to a rather large and long filing cabinet in which, she explained, I could look up books on multiple sclerosis under the letter *M*. She further explained that she could pull a lot of additional research material for me, but due to their closing time within the next few hours, there would be little that she could do for me that day. She inquired if I would like her to proceed on investigating the subject matter, to which I simply answered no. Investigate the subject matter? The subject matter was me, not just what lay in some textbook and research papers.

After searching for about thirty minutes, I collected about five books and found a place to sit. Unfortunately, all the tables were taken, so I went over to the children's section and sat down in a small plastic orange chair at a shortened height table. The children's section was empty; perhaps they were all outside playing.

I lay the books on the table and briefly read over each cover. I opened the first book to its index and fingered down the page to the words *life expectancy*. Without hesitation, I turned to the corresponding page and read the following sentence, almost as if in slow motion, "Average life expectancy upon disease onset is twenty-five years for the male population." I read the same sentence over and over, arguing with myself as to whether or not twenty-five years was a long time, a long enough time for the things I still wanted to do.

I thought about my neighbor, who had recently been diagnosed with ALS or Lou Gehrig's disease. I remember reading an interview in the local paper that he and his wife had given; I don't recall the reason why—probably to raise awareness. I remember making my way through the article when I was suddenly dumbstruck by a comment that they had made regarding their car. They noted that the one thing that probably upset them the most was that they would have to sell their brand-new BMW. I reflected on what a ludicrous and outlandish statement that was. Here was a man who was going to die within three years, physically leave the planet and perhaps the universe, and his main concern was having to sell his brand-new BMW? I showed the article to Michelle for her opinion, and she said that she found it sad because the couple was actually in denial and had not yet grasped the fact that the husband was going to pass away and lose everything he had, that material goods didn't matter anyway.

I remained at the library until closing, absorbing every piece of information I could find. My legs and back were cramped as I sat in that little orange chair, hunched over a child-size table. I found myself wishing to be surrounded by the children who normally sat and read in this section, for their voices and laughter, for the silence to be broken. Silence is not always golden. I was suddenly in a race, a race for knowledge and time. I felt no pity, only concern; all I had to fight this disease with at that time was my intelligence, but would that be enough? Since I had no library card, I could not check out any books, therefore I had to write down all of the information I planned to question the doctor about.

Black or white, true or false, fifty-fifty—I lost the bet either way. As I drove home, I could think of nothing but climbing into bed with Michelle, slipping under cold sheets, and pressing up against her warm body. I knew she would give me my time; I knew she would not question where I had been or what I had been doing. I asked her for so much, she gave me so much, and I gave very little in return.

Prior to leaving the library, I wrote down some of the main topics that I had read about and wanted to talk about in further detail.

1. If twenty-five years of life is the average expectancy for males, what is the maximum life expectancy?
2. How long could I expect to remain ambulatory?
3. How long could I expect to remain employed?
4. How is the bladder affected by MS, and what can be done to help escape?
5. People talk about having the physical sensation of burning or being stuck with pins and needles.

Can you describe this in further detail, and again, what can be done to help this?

6. They say that MS runs a different course for different people. Are there certain things that affect how the course will run? For example, are there special dietary requirements for those with MS?

7. Speaking of life expectancy, can you tell me what the shortest lifespan has been that you have seen? Are there statistics on this subject as well?

8. Do you have any books or special reading material that you can recommend to me?

9. As you know, I have already been diagnosed with, and I'm still suffering from, the effects of optic neuritis. Will my vision ever improve? Do you know of cases where people have gone permanently blind?

10. My fiancée and I plan on having children soon after we are married. Will I experience sexual dysfunction, and if so, is there anything that can be done about it?

11. Is MS hereditary?

These were the main questions that I had, and I felt that if they were answered, that would put my mind somewhat at ease. I didn't know if my mind would ever be permanently at ease, but I knew that I would just have to let life unfold and see.

Diagnosis

May 25, 1995.

Michelle was nothing short of furious with Dr. Hammond. She actually contacted the American Medical Association (AMA) and reported him for leaving my diagnosis on my work voice mail. I never asked her how the call went, partly because I lacked the mental strength to care but mostly because I knew that she could be ferociously defensive of me when the need arose. I'm quite sure that Dr. Hammond suffered some sort of punishment even if it was in the form of a harshly worded reprimand letter from the AMA.

I did follow up once I got back from vacation, but it certainly wasn't with Dr. Hammond. Instead I made an appointment to see his colleague, Dr. Jacobs, the only other doctor my ophthalmologist had given me a business card for. As a side note, at that time, there were not a lot of practicing MS specialists, and these two doctors happened to not only be specialists in the field but also worked close to my home.

As I mentioned, Dr. Jacobs and Dr. Hammond both practiced out of the same office suite. While it didn't seem to bother Michelle all that much, probably because of the letter that she wrote, it bothered me immensely. It wasn't until I was assured by the office nurse that Dr. Hammond was actually out of town for the week that my level of anxiety dropped.

Dr. Jacobs was an extremely nice and pleasant doctor to be around. It was obvious to both Michelle and I that, on some level, Dr. Jacobs had heard about me through Dr. Hammond; we just weren't sure if it was from general word-of-mouth or if Dr. Hammond had received some sort of reprimand from the AMA. I hoped that it wasn't the latter, as I really didn't want to get off on the wrong foot with a second doctor, perhaps the only other doctor in Denver who could help me.

Dr. Jacobs had a traditional office setting for a doctor, nothing out of the ordinary and actually quite boring. For whatever reason, he invited us to sit in his office and not one of the patient's suites; I never asked why. Again, maybe he was making up for his colleague's poor behavior in leaving me a voice-mail diagnosis.

He asked us to forgive him if he had any salad stuck in his teeth as that's what he had for lunch. Michelle giggled, but I didn't find the comment too funny. I was too uptight, and I couldn't stop my leg from shaking (a side effect of MS). He went on about how he was going on a diet and had already lost ten or so pounds while he fumbled to retrieve my MRI results out of the manila packaging that he had filed in one of his personal cabinet drawers under *S* for Seliner.

As I looked around his office, I couldn't help but notice how extreme the differences were between his and my psychologist's office. They were the polar opposites of each other, but then again, I guess that only seemed fitting given their different degrees. Dr. Jacobs's office was painted all white, probably the same contractor's grade of white as the original paint. There was a standard four-by-four-foot window that was heavily tinted because his office, unfortunately for him, faced west, which meant that during the afternoon, and especially in the summertime, his office had to become like an oven. This would explain the cheap plastic fan that sat on his desk, probably from Walmart.

The windows were covered with cheap, white venetian blinds, some of the slats bent and some missing altogether. I assumed that he could find blinds like these in this size for about fifty dollars for the entire kit at the local hardware store. The blinds were pulled up just enough to expose a handle in the window that, when spun, opened the bottom twelve inches of glass, exposing a nice breeze of fresh air through the screen.

His desk was made of a dark wood, real wood, not that fake laminated shit from Best Buy or OfficeMax. The desk fit his office well as it too was small and covered with a thick piece of glass that ran from end to end. On top of that, he had a large monthly calendar that was cluttered with writing and highlighting of different colors. Either he was a busy man in his field or he liked to golf a lot. He also had a picture of his family—two boys and a girl who all seemed to be preteens or thereabouts. His wife was more heavyset than he was; I kind of laughed to myself as I imagined them arguing over dinner about who lost how much weight and what they ate. I wondered for a moment if they had a bet on who would lose the most weight in the shortest time. From all outward appearances, Dr. Jacobs was currently winning the bet, but then again, I had no idea how old the picture was.

He continued rambling about ordinary, mundane things, things I really don't recall. Finally, he began reading the findings from the chief radiologist, and suddenly my ears perked up. He stood up and walked over to his x-ray board while he continued talking. He flipped on the florescent light, stuck up two of the larger MRI slides, and asked us to walk over to him. There was little room to stand as two large plastic plants were set aside the x-ray board, so Michelle decided to stay seated at the doctor's desk.

Was I staring at a picture of my brain? I have to tell you, it is beyond a weird feeling—indescribable is the only word I can use—when you find yourself staring at a crystal-clear picture of your own damaged brain.

Dr. Jacobs went on to tell me about how most of the write-up from the chief radiologist was too technical in nature for his own liking let alone a patient's. Basically, the radiologist had indicated that he found two areas of so-called plaque. Dr. Jacobs explained how exactly the MRI machine detected areas of plaque on the brain and spinal column and what exactly plaque areas were. He indicated that areas of plaque were actually scar tissue that had built up due to the processes of multiple sclerosis.

He said that with MS, the body's own immune system attacks the perfectly healthy myelin sheath that covers the nerves within the body much like plastic covers household electrical wiring for protection. Once the myelin sheath has been stripped away, so to speak, from the nerves, what is left behind is actually scar tissue on the nerves. On an MRI, this scar tissue shows up as white areas on the brain matter or on the spinal column, but it wasn't just limited to these areas alone; scar tissue could be found anywhere in the body by the MRI. Dr. Jacobs went on to show me exactly where on the slides the two areas of plaque were: one on the left hemisphere of my brain and one on my cervical spine.

He finally explained that the reason why scar tissue showed up on an MRI was because the MRI utilized the water molecules within the cells of the body to manipulate them through radio frequency. He said that in areas of the body in which there was no water (that is, scar tissue) the MRI machine cannot manipulate the tissue, and therefore it showed up as white on an MRI scan. "I realize that I have just gone over a lot of technical material in nature, Mike. Do you have any questions for me?" he asked.

"I don't want to sound like I know it all, because I certainly don't, but I recently went to the library and did a lot of research on multiple sclerosis and diagnosis through MRI scans. The information you provided was actually quite helpful and corresponded almost exactly with the information that I found at the library. Thank you," I replied. It was the first time that I had the opportunity to speak in the prior half hour, and it brought a flood of emotions that I did not expect. My speech began to fail me, and a watershed of tears took its place. My bottom lip quivered as I motioned toward the box of tissues on the doctor's desk, asking Michelle if she would please grab me several.

She, too, had begun crying as she watched me help-lessly search for the right words. I had no real questions to ask, only angry statements to make, angry statements that for some reason brought me to tears that I could not stop.

Dr. Jacobs politely interrupted my moment and said that he completely understood how difficult this news was to hear for me and my fiancée. He then nodded his head in understanding, pushing the box of tissues toward Michelle and telling me to take whatever time I needed as we could always schedule another appointment to talk about further details. The palms of my hands hurt as my fingernails dug into them from the fists I had angrily formed.

I struck the top corner of his desk with my left fist, crunching my pinky finger on the thick glass top. "No, no, I've waited too long, and I have a wedding coming up, and both my fiancée and I deserve answers. Not that you are to blame in any way—you have been more than gracious in your approach," I said. "You told me that you understood how difficult this news was to hear, but with all due respect, I doubt that you do, not unless you were in my place." I knew that neither he nor Michelle were aware of my true feelings at the time for, if they were, I would not have been sitting in that meeting on that date. No, I would've been in a hospital for sure.

That first visit was the only time that I almost admitted to Michelle and to my new doctor my true feelings—I wanted to die. But I remained silent. I had stopped crying as the reality of the moment hit me hard. Michelle sobbed as I held her hands, trying, for once, to be the comforter.

Dr. Jacobs suddenly broke the silence. "Mike, there are things that we should try to get through during this appointment; I hope you understand. There are drugs that I could start you on immediately that will help you, especially with the way that I know you are feeling right now and the problems that you are having with your left eye."

"Dr. Jacobs, please understand that I am being completely honest with you when I tell you that I completely trust your judgment. This is what I have needed in a doctor and have not been able to find yet. I'm here today not just to hear a diagnosis, but to begin treatment based on your experience," I said. For the first time, I noticed a smile come across both Michelle's and Dr. Jacobs's faces. Were they, for some reason, concerned that I would refuse treatment? A thought slowly crept into my head; I wondered if Michelle had told him beforehand that I had asked her to keep this a secret from everyone I knew, including my parents.

"Mike, would you be opposed to going on an antidepressant?" he asked.

I had thought of the idea before and had read about them in one of the books in the library, and I had already come to the conclusion that I needed extra help in the form of medication. "No," I replied. "I think it's a good idea. Mark this down as drug number one, day number one of countless others. This drug was to help me with depression. I know I need the help. I don't really know much about multiple sclerosis with the exception of what I read in the library the other afternoon and what you've told me now. I wrote down a list of questions based on what I had read, and I would greatly appreciate if you would address them for me and my fiancée. Would you mind doing that?"

"Certainly not, Mike. That's what I'm here for. I'm glad to hear you ask me this," he replied. "Do you have an actual list of questions that you want to go over? If so, please start asking, and I'll do my best to answer them. If there's something you don't understand in my responses, just stop me and let me know, OK?"

"OK, I'll just start going down my list. First off, I read that I have approximately twenty-five years to live, based on my diagnosis date. Is this statistic still accurate?" I asked.

"Twenty-five years to live?" he asked. His question was followed by slight laughter. "Mike, I apologize. My laughter is not directed at you; it's directed at the obviously outdated material that you read. My God, you must have been scared to death when you read that. Multiple sclerosis is not in and of itself a death sentence. Multiple sclerosis is a chronic disease, meaning that, while it progressively gets worse over time, it can be treated. You are not going to die from multiple sclerosis, OK? Are we straight on that point? This is very important."

I didn't know what to think. His answer threw me for a loop, a big loop that I could not jump off of. A smile crept across my face, and I actually felt lightheaded, as this news changed everything for me.

"I'm not sure what to tell you, Dr. Jacobs. I honestly thought that I was going to die within twenty-five years and I was really pondering what I was going to do in the short amount of time I thought I had left. Now that you've told me that I'm not going to die, I almost feel as though I want to leave right now and go celebrate, as crazy as that may sound," I replied.

"That doesn't sound crazy at all, and I think that if I were in your position and were to hear what I just heard, I would probably go out and celebrate too." Dr. Jacobs had a grin on his face that was truly honest.

I looked over at Michelle and squeezed her hand even tighter. She reciprocated and asked me poignantly what I wanted to do.

I told both Dr. Jacobs and her that I wanted to go through the rest of the questions that I had and that we could celebrate this news later that evening.

"OK, moving on, how long can I expect to remain ambulatory?" I asked.

Dr. Jacobs responded, "That question's a little more difficult for me or any doctor to answer. In reality, the answer relies on many different factors, some of which are intangibles and others that are tangible, such as with the ABC medications. These medications are used to help lessen the number of relapses that you may experience. These relapses are also called exacerbations. On average, the ABC medications can reduce the amount of exacerbations that a patient may experience anywhere from thirty-three percent up to forty-four percent."

Dr. Jacobs continued, "Mike, you have what we call relapsing-remitting MS, and our current treatment goal is to keep you ambulatory and working for as long as possible. Since you have been doing some research, maybe you came across mention of the ABC treatment medications?"

"Yes, Avonex, Betaseron, and Copaxone," I replied.

"Yes, and out of those three, Avonex is currently showing the most promise in treating relapsing-remitting MS," he said. "What's nice about Avonex is that it's only a once-a-week shot that is injected into the muscle tissue of your thigh on either leg or on your buttocks. You can either give yourself the shot, or you can come into the office, and the nurse can deliver the shot for you. It all depends on your tolerance level in dealing with shots," he said.

"Currently, all I can tell you is that I don't foresee myself having any problems giving myself a once-a-week shot. I'm not squeamish about shots nor am I squeamish about blood," I replied.

"OK, that's good. Then I'll have my nurse set up a regular shipment of medications to your home address. We do have some medication here in the office, and with your approval, I'd like to give you a shot today so we can get the ball rolling. Does that sound like an acceptable game plan?" he asked.

"Yes, I'd like to get started on this as soon as possible. I assume that your nurse can walk me through how to deliver the shot?" I asked.

"Sure. She has plenty of experience in this area, so not to worry," he said.

"All right, moving on. People talk about having the physical sensation of burning or being stuck with pins and needles. Can you describe this in further detail, and again what can be done to help this?" I asked.

"Well Mike, what you're describing really lies at the crux of multiple sclerosis and one of the mechanisms by which it works. What happens when you're feeling these sensations is that you are actually having what is called an exacerbation. This is where the disease itself is actually alive and active. What is occurring inside your nervous system (which includes the brain and spinal column) is that your body's own defense mechanism is attacking the protective sheath that wraps each nerve. The protective sheath is called the myelin sheath. Once the sheath has been destroyed, the raw nerve is then exposed to the body, where it is free to come in contact with other nerves, muscle tissue, skin, etc. When you feel these electrical shocks or pinpricks, the exposed nerve is coming in contact with other body parts. The medication that we discussed earlier tries to prevent or slow down the number of exacerbations that your body experiences, thus reducing the amount of scar tissue that you are left with in your nervous system. There's an old drug on the market that works wonderfully for helping to prevent the pain associated with an exacerbation, and it's called Neurontin." Mark this down as drug number three, my first pain medication.

"Does this help to explain what an exacerbation is for you, Mike?" he asked.

"Yeah, thank you. That was an excellent explanation and one that really put things into perspective for me," I said.

"OK, what other questions do you have on your plate?" he asked.

"They say that MS runs a different course for different people. Are there certain things that affect how the course will run? For example, are there special dietary requirements for those with MS?" I asked.

"I get asked this question all the time, and the easiest answer that I can give you is, no. While you'll read claims about new dietary breakthroughs about every month, I would tell you not to bother with them. Make sense?" he asked.

"Yes it does, and that's kinda what I figured you were about to say but I had to ask it," I said. "OK, last major question for me, and then we can move on. My fiancée and I plan on having children soon after we are married. Will I experience sexual dysfunction, and if so, is there anything that can be done about it?

"Good question, Mike. While I cannot predict the future for certain, there is a high probability that you will experience sexual dysfunction in some form at some point in your life. The good news is that there are now plenty of ED medications on the market to help men who are experiencing problems. With that said, I don't think you have too much to worry about," he said.

"OK—that's all I have right now except for some other minor things. Thank you for taking the time to go over this with me," I said. "The only other immediate concern that I have is in regard to my left eye and my inability to see properly."

"Our options for treatment regarding your eye are a little more narrowed. Optic neuritis is basically a condition of the eye in which severe inflammation is occurring simultaneously with the myelin sheath being attacked by your body's immune system. In essence, you are experiencing an exacerbation involving your optic nerve. Since you are just starting treatment to prevent further exacerbations with the Avonex, we can only really try to stop the severe inflammation that is also playing a major role in your ability to see properly.

"What we normally do in this case is start a three- to four-day course of very strong steroids. Because the steroids can have side effects relative to your heart rate and insulin level, you will have to be hospitalized for this time frame just so we can keep an eye on you, no pun intended. Is there any way that you can be admitted to the hospital today?" he asked.

"Yes, I really can't think of anything more important than starting the treatment for this, based on what you have said. Is this something that your nurse can help set up for me also?" I asked.

"Sure, I'll get her working on that right away, and in the meantime, I ask that you stop by your house and pick up your essentials, such as toiletries and so on, and then return my office when you're ready. Do you have any questions?" he asked.

"No, I think I understand everything, and if I have any questions, I'll just give your nurse a call," I said.

I felt a huge relief after leaving the doctor's office that day. Dr. Jacobs was a straight shooter. I had a lot of personality traits in common with him, and for that, I was grateful. I was also grateful to have confirmation that the drug I was on showed the best benefits in treating relapsing-remitting MS patients. The drug Avonex was proven to cut down on new lesions (or relapses) by nearly 44 percent.

I knew Michelle wanted to talk with me on the way back to our apartment; however, she also knew that I wanted to mull things over in my head. I needed time alone, time that I knew would come once she boarded her flight back home, which was later that evening. She asked if I wanted her to cancel her flight. It was a loaded question that came with all the trimmings—if I said no, it would simply be too unfair to her and her feelings, and if I said yes, I knew that I would have someone I trusted with me for at least another day, another weekend. "Yes, Michelle, yes, I would like you to stay," I replied.

"Thank you," she said quietly.

PSYCHOTHERAPY

April 13, 2007.

"You seem a lot happier today than I've seen you in a while," Bob said.

"I'm not quite sure if happier is the word I would choose," I said.

"What word would you choose to use?" Bob asked.

"I'd like to go back and talk about the period in my life when I was diagnosed," I said.

"That's fine. Go ahead," Bob said.

"Anyway, I'm not really sure if there's a word for it; it's more of an emotion. I had just been diagnosed by my neurologist with relapsing-remitting multiple sclerosis," I said. "It's not that I felt happy, but I guess you could say that I felt glad, oddly enough. I felt like a weight had been lifted off my chest. That whole time, I was walking around thinking I had a brain tumor, only to find out that it's your garden-variety MS. Granted, I had no idea what was in store for me, but listen to me: you're right.

I was happier than I was. I was happier now that I knew I didn't have a brain tumor, but I wasn't happy to know that I had MS. I guess the whole situation was just anti-climactic in a sense.

"I don't really know how to describe it. Hell, I don't even know how to describe how I'm feeling right now. What I need is your professional help. I need therapy. Can you help me with that? Can you help me with the conundrum that I'm in?" Christ, I felt like I just jumped down the fucking rabbit hole without a safety harness. Hell, at that point, I'd have settled for a bungee cord. At least that way, I could bounce back up and out. Was that a reference to bipolar disorder?

"Mike, we'll work through this together. I'm not going anywhere; I'm here to help you for as long as you need it, and hopefully you understand that by now," he said.

"Yeah, I understand. I trust you, Bob, it's…well, just look at me. For the first time, I'm tearless; I'm emotionless. Is this a problem? Should it be a problem? What are your thoughts right now?" I asked.

"What I think is that you've been through a hell of a lot, and your mind, just like anyone else's, is having trouble processing everything at once," he said. "What you need to do, what we need to do, rather, is develop a game plan for not just what you have already been through but what else may possibly happen to you. What we need to do is eliminate the surprises in your life. It's the surprises or the gotchas that are causing you great strife, and we need to try to eliminate those as best we can."

I began to cry long before he started speaking. The tears were back. All the stress had been building for so long, and I felt like I had no real release mechanism, nowhere to go in private to try to process everything I had been through. Bob knew that my happiness was nothing short of a small sense of relief from the constant bombardment of grief that my mind was under. I was close to a complete meltdown; another Three Mile Island incident.

"Can we talk about your then fiancée for a bit, Mike?" he asked. "Had you talked to her yet about your diagnosis?"

I stared out the window for a while. Again, I found myself lost, staring at someone else moving in their belongings into one of the storage garages across the street. I don't know why, but it seemed ridiculous that my mind was so preoccupied by someone storing their belongings. I never mentioned anything to Bob about it as I was sure that he would have a long-winded reason for why I was so preoccupied by it, and I didn't feel like listening to it.

They were a couple, probably in their midthirties, with two young boys who were unloading a wood-paneled, lime-green station wagon and trailer. The station wagon was old and rusted—I was surprised that it was still running from the amount of oil it was burning—and the trailer had a large blue tarp tied down over their belongings. Were these all of the belongings that the family owned?

Their younger boys mainly ran around the gated parking lot while the couple cut the twine off the tarp and removed it from the trailer. The scenario seemed sad in some manner. It was sad that everything the family had owned might have been in the back of that trailer. Did their kids understand?

"Mike. Mike, are you with me?" Bob asked.

"Yes, Bob, sorry, you caught me daydreaming," I said. "To answer your question, yes, my fiancée was aware of the entire situation and what I had been through," I replied.

"And do you mind me asking what her response was?" he asked.

"She was upset by the whole incident, yet very supportive of me and the situation in general. She repeated our wedding vows, which brought me some relief. Actually a lot of relief," I said. "The bad part, however, was that it happened during our vacation to Las Vegas. I call it a vacation, but it turned out to be anything but."

Bob pressed on, asking, "What was so bad about the vacation? What happened exactly?"

I replied that my neurologist had left my diagnosis on my work voice mail.

"You mean to tell me that he asked you to come into his office so he could speak with you, correct?" he asked.

"No, he actually gave me the diagnosis multiple sclerosis on my work voice mail," I said.

"So he never talked to you in person?" he asked.

"Nope. And he even had my mobile number to call me. I had it with me the whole time, and he never left a single fucking message, which is what was so confusing about the matter. I don't ever remember giving him my work voice mail, unless he called my work phone number directly and got it from there," I said.

Bob said, "That is absolutely the most ludicrous, unbelievable story I have ever heard in my professional career. As a matter of fact, I'd go so far as to say that I've never heard anything like it. Is he still your doctor?"

"Oh, no," I replied. "My wife, who was my fiancée at the time, made sure of that. She actually wrote a letter to the AMA complaining about what he had done, but if they did anything, I never heard about it. I never received a response letter from the AMA."

"I'm sorry that happened to you, Mike. Rest assured that I would never do anything like that to you or to any of my patients. Can I ask who you are now seeing, just for my records?"

"Sure," I replied. "I'm seeing a Dr. Jacobs. Unfortunately, he practices out of the same office suite as Dr. Hammond does, but I've come to learn that multiple sclerosis is not a highly practiced specialty within neurology, and these are the only two doctors relatively close to my house. Besides, based on the letter my wife wrote, I don't think that I'll be bumping into him anytime soon."

I wasn't looking directly at Bob, but I could tell that he was staring at me from behind his desk. I think he felt a certain amount of comfort behind that desk as that's where he could be found during most of our sessions.

"What else can I help you with, Bob? I know there's more on your mind, something you want to ask me maybe, but you're afraid?" I asked. I found my question rather harsh and uncalled for after I had asked it. There was a change building inside me again, and it all centered on the rage I felt, rage like when I had dealt with

Dr. Hammond. I found that I was no longer pushing things to the back of my mind, locking them up in my special vault. That's where I put memories I didn't want to deal with and memories I most likely would not need to retrieve for a long time, if ever.

"I know I said early on in our meeting that you seemed happier than usual to me. I now stand corrected and owe you an apology," he said.

I personally didn't think that he owed me anything, and I also didn't think that I owed him anything, especially not in the form of an apology. Bob was my therapist. He was a professional, and he knew the risks associated with each patient.

"Your wife is a strong person in your relationship; do you recognize her as such?" he asked.

"Can you tell me what you're trying to get at, Bob? I'm sorry, but I'm not quite sure I understand the point you're trying to make," I said.

"Well, you have been seeing her for quite some time, and yet your relationship still seems as strong as ever. You seem to confide in her quite a bit, and she also seems to protect you from a lot of the things that you have to do deal with. Would you consider those to be fair statements, Mike?" he asked.

"No doubt, Bob. I love her and can confide in you that quite honestly I do not see any faults in her. But I ask that you please not say that she somehow protects me from a lot of the things that I have to deal with. No one protects me from the things I go through except for me." I felt strongly about this situation in my life, and in general, no one had protected me or helped me along this path except for me. I don't feel that anyone else should receive credit for protecting or helping me, with maybe the exception of my parents.

Bob fell quiet, and I guess he chose not to respond for whatever reason. I wanted to come across strong because I wanted to put an end to this perception of protection. Hopefully I had done just that.

I was staring out the window again, but the family in the lime-green station wagon was gone. I looked around for someone else dumping off or picking up their belongings, but the storage lot was empty. I heard Bob at his desk, shuffling through his notepad probably for the next topic that he wanted to discuss. What happened? Was he losing his touch? Usually the flow of his therapy was quite congruent, but something had interrupted his normal path.

Oh, well, I didn't feel like talking for the moment anyway, and I knew Bob would come up with a topic rather quickly. In the meantime, I continued my scouting mission of the storage facility across the street. I had a perfect viewpoint from as we were on the third floor, and the entire storage facility was built of slab on grade construction (the entire building was single-story). One thing that struck me was the inordinate amount of security that completely surrounded the facility and kept guard. If you were to remove all of the signs from the storage complex and ask someone who was new to this country what was stored there, I'm sure that person would reply that somehow money played a role. Maybe it was a printing facility or a repository of sorts.

In any event, the entire facility was surrounded by what had to be an eight-foot high wrought-iron fence covered with razor wire at the top. There was absolutely no way anyone could get in through the fencing system. I even imagined that they had electrified the fencing system itself, which would deal a lethal blow to whoever was dumb enough to try to enter. In between the fence runs, large concrete-brick structures helped to tie the fencing systems together. On top of these brick structures sat a high-definition camera looking around the entire lot. I guess it would have been kind of reassuring to me had I wanted to store items there. At the same time, I was a little creeped out as I wondered what type of working-class neighborhood I was in.

Bob interrupted my daydreaming again with a light cough followed by, "Excuse me, Mike, can we talk a bit about what you did prior to being diagnosed? If memory serves me well, I believe you told me that you headed off to the library the day after you got back from your vacation in Vegas, is that correct?" he asked. "You told me that you grabbed a handful of books in the library and hoped you'd find an open seat in or near the children's section. Is all that correct?"

"Yep, except I wasn't hoping to sit in the children section, it just happened to be the only seating available. Other than that, you nailed it." I asked him what he wanted to know in particular, I was also beginning to wonder if Bob was getting used to my regular daydreaming spells.

"Why the library? Why not the Internet?" he asked.

"Well, it seemed to me that, and this is just my opinion, most of the things on the Internet are junk in nature and really shouldn't be trusted. Besides that, I cannot do a single search on a single item without something pornographic in nature popping up. It's really kind of aggravating."

Bob laughed a bit, I think about how the Internet was full of pornographic material. "Tell me, Mike, when you had those books in your hand, what was the first thing that you had decided look up or find out about multiple sclerosis?"

"Interesting question, and I remember it clearly. I wanted to know how long I had to live," I said.

"So you thought that multiple sclerosis had a death sentence tied to it, and you wanted to know how much longer you had to live?"

"Correct. I wouldn't come to find out until later at my appointment with Dr. Jacobs that multiple sclerosis does not carry a death sentence, and that most people with MS usually die from other opportunistic diseases or illnesses that may strike when the patient is having an exacerbation," I said. "So I guess I learned three things on that day. One is you can't trust the information on the Internet; two, the books of my local library are outdated; and three, MS does not carry a death sentence, especially not in today's age."

Bob asked, "What did the books at the library have to say as far as length of time to death?"

The question irked me, and I found myself squirming and not wanting to answer it, but I was too tired not to. "It said that I had twenty-five years to live, on average, upon diagnosis," I said.

"I can only imagine how panicked and upset you were in that moment. You were by yourself?" Bob said.

"Yeah, you're right. I was panicked to say the least. You know what I thought of when I read that sentence,

Bob? I tried to rationalize that twenty-five years was plenty of time to do the things that I wanted to do. How fucking crazy is that?" I said.

"I don't think it's crazy at all. It's just how the brain works. In that moment, you were in what is called survival mode; it was your fight-or-flight instinct. You could have run to avoid the situation, or you could have stayed to fight it on some level. Your brain, probably because of your intelligence level, decided to stay and fight, to try to come to some sort of understanding with this disease called MS and whether you had the time that you wanted to complete the things that you obviously felt still need completing," Bob said. "Can you see how this is true? Does it make sense to you now?"

"Yeah, it does. I can see what you're trying to say, and I do agree with it."

Bob asked, "Do you recall the next thing you decided to research?"

I stared at the ornate design of his throw rug, which had obviously been produced outside of the country. At least I hoped so; I did not want the throw rug to be another mirage of the things that Bob had either once done or the places he had once traveled to. I immediately asked him where he got the throw rug, as I found its design quite ornate.

A smile quickly came across Bob's face, and I had the sensation of relief as I knew what he was going to say next. "Believe it or not, my friend and I went to India for vacation one year, New Delhi to be exact, or at least that's where we started. We actually spent nearly a month there, but when you're traveling abroad and trying to do some sightseeing. you just about need to take a month's reprieve. I bought the rug at a factory that exports them to the United States, but you can get them in New Delhi for pennies on the dollar. The most expensive part was having it shipped back home, but I still came out ahead, as it would have cost me a couple thousand more had I bought it in the States." Bob. said. "Sorry to ramble on so much about the rug, but there is quite a lengthy story behind it."

"I'm sure there is, and from what you've already told me, it sounds quite interesting," I said.

"Well, Mike, we've already gone over, and for that I apologize, but in our next session I do want to talk about work and marriage, OK?" he asked.

"That sounds fine. Thanks for listening," I said.

LOVE AND MARRIAGE

June 1, 1995.

I'm not sure why, but I pushed off marriage for the longest time. It's not that I was not in love with my fiancée; I think it was a feeling that maybe there was something or someone else out there for me that I couldn't quite put my finger on. I already felt like my life was over with the diagnosis.

I'm sure everyone has found themselves in similar situations at one time or another. It has nothing to do with who we are or with our feelings for others; it's a lack of something within us. It's hard to describe in words; only those who know truly understand. I needed a swift kick in the bottom, otherwise I knew I would lose the love of my life, and that was something that I had no intention of going through. I received that kick one evening in what was probably the shortest, yet most important, conversation I ever had, and one I believe I deserved the most.

Michelle walked into my den one evening after work, pointed to her ring finger, and said, "Do you see this?"

"Yes, it's a finger," I said.

"Correct, and more precisely, it's my ring finger," she said.

"And your point is?" I asked.

"We've been dating for close to ten years now, and unless there is one big freaking ring on this finger within the next month, I'm moving on! I love you very much, Michael, but my eggs won't wait forever," she said.

Ring? Eggs? There were two—check that, three things I remember after that conversation, three things I will never forget. The first was the word *ring*, or, more precisely, *big freaking ring*. Michelle already had a ring on her finger, but apparently, that ring was not big enough! The second was the word *egg*, more precisely *eggs*, the plural form, which implied she wanted more than one child and did not put a limit on the number of children. The third was the sound of a biplane flying a banner around my empty head that simply read, "Game Over."

While sitting in the dark, staring out the window at the nearby foothills of the Rocky Mountains, I slowly rolled my chair up to my computer and did a little research. I wanted to see if there were any statistics on how long marriages actually lasted. I thought it only fair, as we had been seeing each other for nearly ten years and had not only loved each other very much but had few issues during that entire time. Michelle and I were more than just in love; we were best friends. We enjoyed each other's hobbies and especially enjoyed being DINKs (dual income, no kids). There's definitely something to be said for being able to spend all the time alone that you wanted with the one you loved without the worry of interruption or money, especially when you're living in a city like Denver.

What I found shocked me, and it has since become a mantra of mine that I tell all those willing to listen. I tell them not to discourage them from getting married, but so that they understand that marriage is work. Over a seven-year period, you have a better chance of winning a coin toss than staying married. That's right! Fifty-two percent of married couples will be divorced within a seven-year period. While I wasn't sure that I liked the odds, it certainly wasn't a conversation I was ever going to have with then fiancée.

June 15, 1996.

Our wedding day finally arrived. It was a surprisingly hot, muggy day in mid-June; usually the really hot, humid summer months don't come until the middle to end of July in Missouri. Thunderstorms were forecasted due to the extreme heat, but they seemed to be holding out as we made our way from the parking lot into the cool, air-conditioned church. The church itself was not of my choosing. I would have preferred to get married where I grew up, in Affton.

Yes, in case you're wondering, this is the same Affton where actor John Goodman grew up. I still recall hearing stories about how he would come back from time to time during our school picnics and devour some of the most delicious barbecue that groups of drunken men slaved over from seven in the morning until midnight.

However, which church we used was not my choice to make, and I don't remember putting up too much of a fight about it. I was just happy to be getting married. I had grown so fond of the idea of being together forever with the one I loved so much that little else seemed to matter.

Once inside the church, the groomsmen and I made our way back to the rectory, where we were able to have some drinks and change into our tuxedos. As I was getting into mine, one of my groomsmen told me that my mother was out in the church looking for me. I hadn't seen either my mother or father on the way in, so I asked him to bring them back to the rectory so I could say hi.

When my parents entered the rectory and I had the opportunity to see them, I was completely astonished. My mother looked absolutely stunning in a brand-new, full-length blue silk dress with a corsage. I had heard earlier that my father had lost some weight but was absolutely shocked when I saw the new him. He had lost close to eighty pounds and looked about ten years younger! It really was one of the highlights of my wedding to see them both together looking so good and appearing so happy. I was so proud of my father; he had even stopped smoking, which really put a smile on my face. We had tried to get him to stop for decades.

After we took a few pictures together, they had to leave the rectory as I needed to get ready for the wedding.

The rectory was spacious, clean, and neatly adorned with what I could only imagine was a collection of expensive miscellaneous souvenirs and gifts that the priests had been given over the years and displayed on numerous oak shelves. A note from the family who donated each gift was placed beside it, and after reading a few, it was apparent that these gifts were given to the priests by the couples they married. Odd that I had forgotten such a simple act of kindness, but I was sure that Michelle had taken care of this small token—at least I prayed she had.

As the groomsmen were changing, I sat on a small foldout chair next to one of two floor-to-ceiling windows that let in an immense amount of natural light—so much light that lamps were not needed during the daytime. There were no curtains or sheers or blinds to cover the windows. I looked out into the parking lot and watched friends I knew and some I had never met make their way from their cars across what I imagined was a hot blacktop surface, giving off the kind of heat that would penetrate the souls of thick leather shoes and make feet bake and sweat. It was a short walk in any event, and I knew they would soon be relieved by the air conditioner that was working overtime to keep the interior at a cool seventy degrees.

Every couple of minutes, I stared down at the watch on my wrist, ensuring that I would not be late for the most important event in my life. Why was I even worried about being late? There was nowhere I could go. Even if I wanted to make a run for it, I was sure I'd be tackled halfway to my car.

One of my groomsmen, Mike, offered me a shot of whiskey, a gesture that for seemed sacrilege inside His house. Mike looked at me with a funny smirk on his face and said, "I'm sure you had enough of this last night to last you a lifetime, but from the look on your face, you need this."

I did everything I could to prevent the image of me falling backward off the altar while exchanging vows from creeping into my mind.

"You also need to know that everything is going to be fine, so stop worrying. I can see the sweat near your hairline," he said.

My best man, Tom, decided he wanted a shot also, and then it was only minutes before all the guys had shot glasses filled and raised in salute to me and my wife-to-be. The shot went down easily; my gut put up no resistance. I guess it had done that enough last night and early this morning. It did its job, though; it helped me relax while improving my spirits and dispelling the worry. This truly was the best day of my life.

Again I sat down and stared out the window to see how full the parking lot was. My own wedding day, and the only thing I could think of was how many people were going to be in attendance when there was only one person who truly mattered. I suddenly noticed the strong smell of incense burning and assumed that the priest must have been blessing the altar.

My best man drew up a seat next to me and looked outside at the people still making their way in. He jokingly asked, "What if nobody shows up?"

"No, I don't see that happening. I'm more worried about where they're all going to park," I said. To my surprise, the parking lot was full, and people were now being forced to park out on the adjoining street. It would only be a matter of minutes before the priest decided to start the ceremony.

"You feel good, Mr. Seliner?" Tom asked jokingly.

"I feel great, and I want to thank you again for being my best man," I said.

"I wouldn't have it any other way, my friend," Tom said.

At two o'clock, our scheduled start time, the priest came back into the rectory and said that he wanted to wait another fifteen minutes as people were still making their way into the church. My heart raced again. I thought about the lines I had committed to memory and went over them in my head one more time. With my eyes closed, the priest gently grabbed my right hand, waking me from thought, and told me not to worry or be concerned. If I got lost along the way, all I had to do was whisper to him the key word *help*. He laughed quietly and said that I needed to remember that this was the most important day of my life and that messing up or forgetting a few words would not be the end of the world. "We're in God's house, Michael, and you need to place your faith in Him."

At two fifteen, the ceremony commenced, and both groomsmen and bridesmaids made their way out to the altar, where the priest was awaiting us. I remember being the main attraction at an event for the first time ever. I felt all eyes on me at the moment. I gazed at all the familiar faces in the crowd and was overcome with joy. It meant so much for me to have all my friends and family surrounding me on that special day. That day in which I knew no bond could be broken. I had a grin from ear to ear that could not be wiped away. I felt happiness that knew no bounds. Yes, good does exist, and on this special day, nothing could touch us. I felt higher than I had ever been in my life, and I was in the house of my Lord. For this, I thanked Him in my mind in my own way.

"Wedding March" began playing, and at the end of the long center aisle, the heavy wooden doors were pushed open, revealing my beautiful bride. She was nothing short of stunning. The entire church turned in their seats to see her; some stood to see and photograph her. I made my way down three sets of marble stairs that completely encompassed the altar to meet my bride.

I could only imagine what was going through my soon-to-be father-in-law's mind. He was symbolically handing off his only daughter, trusting her to no one but me. He stood toe-to-toe with me, gave me a hug, and whispered, almost begging for one simple thing. "Please take care of my daughter, Michael. I love you like a son."

I stared for a moment at my bride; her smile was so bright, and she beamed with honest happiness. I took all those moments in as I knew they would be short-lived. We interlocked arms and walked up the steps to the priest, the master of ceremonies. My best man, Tom, gave me a pat of reassurance on my right arm. I had no doubts; this was our moment.

"Michael, do you take Michelle to be your wife? Do you promise to be true to her in good times and in bad, in sickness and in health, to love her and honor her all the days of your life?" the priest asked.

I paused momentarily as my eyes met those of Michelle's aunt, Mary Jane. I noticed for the first time that she had been silently crying and was staring intently at me and smiling. Those words that the priest had just spoken to me made me think deeply of the love that I had for my fiancée and how everything was about to change with two spoken words. I could feel the crowd that had gathered within the church that day was hanging on my very breath. I smiled back at Mary Jane, and then looked deeply into Michelle's eyes and said, "I do."

"Michelle, do you take Michael to be your husband? Do you promise to be true to him in good times and in bad, in sickness and in health, to love him and honor him all the days of your life?" the priest asked.

"I do," she said.

Newly married and living in a new house, we were pretty much on track with things, including our careers. However, there were one or two things missing, like kids. We had discussions about having kids on and off for the past year, and my wife was a definite proponent of having them. I, on the other hand, was a little more skittish as I could not get out of my mind the fact that my neurologist had indicated that the risk of having children who could later develop MS was eight times greater than for the normal population. Michelle tried to convince me that like so much of what I had read, this information might be obsolete also. There was also no confirmation that MS was hereditary, so for us, it was pretty much a crapshoot, and she and I knew how much I didn't care for gambling. To add insult to injury, I don't think I could have ever forgiven myself had any of my children developed MS. I'm not quite sure why Michelle seemed to have so much of an easier time with the whole scenario; perhaps her faith was simply greater than mine. This discussion would need to be tabled for later.

Not only did we have this issue to deal with, but I also knew that I finally needed to open up and talk to my family about being diagnosed with the disease. Too many years had gone by without me telling them, and I believed they were still suspicious about our trip to Las Vegas a few years back. I needed to contact my mother and father and deliver the news that would probably devastate them.

I sat on the floor of our family room with the television on low, holding the phone loosely in my sweaty hand. I was sick to my stomach, and despite the many times I swallowed down another Tums, I still received no relief. As I went to make that first phone call, I immediately hung the receiver up; it was like I was making that initial phone call to my neurologist all over again.

Finally, I managed to build up the nerve and stay on the line. I knew my mother would answer the phone, and I tried to picture what she may be doing at seven thirty in the evening. She'd be playing games on her computer while watching TV, I thought. Given the circumstances, I knew it might take a while for her to process the information, but there simply was no good way to deliver bad news.

"Hello?" she said.

"Mom, it's me, Michael," I said.

"Oh, hi, honey, how you doing?" she asked.

"Not too bad, but I need to talk to you about a serious matter. Do you and Dad have a few minutes?" I asked.

"Michael, what's the matter?" she asked.

"Something has developed, and I think it's best that both you and Dad are on the line while I'm talking to you. Is that OK?" I asked.

"OK, hang on a minute, and I'll go get your father," she said. "OK, can you hear me? We're both on the line now."

"Hi, Dad. Long time no see. You doing OK?" I said.

"Yeah, I'm doing OK. Is everything all right with you?" he asked.

"Well, that's kind of the reason that I'm calling you guys tonight. I've been putting off this discussion for far too long, and I hope that you can forgive me for doing so. In the summer of 1995, I was diagnosed with a disease called multiple sclerosis. It's a chronic disease that affects the central nervous system and one that is different for each individual. There is no cure for it, but there are medications available to slow its progression."

The television volume in the background was turned down as my mother was apparently now beginning to process what it was that was affecting her son. I don't know why exactly, but I recall feeling sad for her and wanting to be there in person.

"Michael, is this something that you can die from? Please tell the truth; we're not mad at you about not telling us sooner," my mother said.

"Well, I'll put it to you like my neurologist put it to me…I won't die from multiple sclerosis itself. People with the disease usually end up dying from other opportunistic diseases such as pneumonia," I responded.

"Have you been taking medications this whole time? I mean, I haven't noticed any difference in you over the past several years. I'm assuming that you've had the disease for some time before they diagnosed it," my father said.

"Good point, dad. Since being diagnosed, I have been on a drug by the name of Avonex, and it's supposed to cut down on future outbreaks by up to forty-four percent, which is quite a bit when you think about the fact that the average person diagnosed with relapsing-remitting MS has an exacerbation (as they are called) or outbreak once every two years. I'm also on a handful of other drugs to help control muscle rigidity and whatnot. Right now, I'm doing fine. I'm feeling fine, and I've been this way since diagnosis but that's key. I have actually had the disease since probably 1992, but with the symptoms being so mundane, I never sought the help of a neurologist because I never thought anything was wrong.

"This disease can go a multitude of different ways, so there's no point in worrying about it too much. As my neurologist said it best, I just pretty much have to let the disease run its course. He'll deal with the exacerbations if and when they come up," I said. "I know I've told you guys a lot of information in a short amount of time, and I'm sure that more than anything you're probably just worried at this point, and I don't blame you one bit. I can't begin to apologize for not telling you sooner. I was not trying to hide anything from either of you; I was just trying my best to keep you from having to worry."

"Honey, you know that we both love you and will support you as a much as we possibly can, OK?" my mother said.

"I know you do, Mom, and I love the both of you very much. I'll be coming back to town sometime within the next three months, and then I'll be able to come over and talk to you in further detail about the disease itself. In the meantime, you can go on to the Internet and do a Google search for the National Multiple Sclerosis Society. They have plenty of information there that you can print out and start reading up on. When I come back to town, I'll bring more material with me that will teach you everything you want to know about the disease and then some. Does that sound like a game plan?" I asked.

"Yeah, honey, it will be great to be able to see you again, and I'll go on the Internet like you suggested. We both love you very much, OK? You take care and call us back soon," my mother said.

I could picture my father comforting my mother as she cried. I prayed to God that this was not the case, but I knew how I would feel if one of my kids were to tell me that they had such a disease. What could I do to ease her grief? Not too much. I had held out for years, and sooner or later the truth had to come out. More damage would have been done by continuing to keep them in the dark. The call was over, and Michelle asked me how things had gone. All I could say was fine. I was completely emotionless for the first time in a long time. I guess delivering the news was anticlimactic; maybe I would feel differently later, but for now, I simply felt nothing at all.

MEMORIES

October 9, 1999.

I had not seen my young nephew in several months, and my wife and I thought it would be a good idea for a break back to St. Louis to see our families. When I finally did see him, I don't believe that he recognized me or even noticed me walking in between the television and him. For his own good reasons, he simply sat there in the middle of the family-room floor, playing video games by himself. Michelle headed off to the back bedroom where my sister slept to check in on her. Debbie had called, knowing that we were in town and had asked that we stop by with the few items she asked us to pick up for her.

I chose to remain behind for the moment to sit down on the floor next to my young nephew and decided for to ask him if he knew who I was. I tried to see my sister whenever I was in town, but I lived over 350 miles away, and taking the time off work and making the drive was not something that was too conducive to my work schedule.

Debbie lived with Vincent down in the city in a third-floor apartment that looked like it had been built in the early 1960s. The paint on the walls looked original, and I know for certain that all of the ornate woodwork around the windows and doorways was. It was a two-bedroom apartment, but Vincent had his own bed in his mother's room. His own room had not really been decorated, and it was apparent that he spent most of his time with his mother, as most of his toys were in her bedroom. It was kind of strange in that her bedroom was one of the largest rooms in the house. She had added her own personal touch of decorating, which meant that the room was littered with memorabilia from the past, like black-and-white movie posters and framed photographs. She had a lot more friends than I was aware of.

Again, you could immediately see her love for the actor Vincent Price. I grew up never really understanding her infatuation with him or the past in general. I just remember her talking about how good of an actor she thought he was and how she loved the show that he hosted. I can't remember the name of it off the top of my head—I think it was *House of Usher*, but I could be wrong. In any event, he was plastered everywhere. There was no free space on her walls.

St. Louis has the equivalent of Chicago's *L*; however, it's called the Metro Link. The Metro Link mainly runs from St. Louis County (the suburbs) into the city and ends on the East Side, which is actually located in Illinois. It just so happened that the city constructed an elevated portion of the Metro directly in back of her apartment, and while not nearly as loud as the *L*, it still made a racket as it went by on its regular thirty-minute schedule. In Debbie's room, the sound was impossible to escape; however, she was quite immune to it. When I brought it up, she simply shrugged her shoulders.

When Vincent was in her room, he constantly ran to look out at the Metro, as you could see the passengers inside even at night. He seemed to get a kick out of it, and he giggled every time one went by.

There were no cats to be seen anywhere in the apartment, but it was obvious that at one time, cats had roamed around, apparently using parts of the apartment as a litter box. It was sad to think that they once had pets that Vincent had loved, but since Debbie couldn't take care of them anymore, they had either been given away or become outdoor animals. I'm not sure why, but with every passing year, I became more sentimental and more protective of my family.

Every window was decorated with long, white flowing sheers; there were no drapes in the apartment. The kitchen was an absolute disaster with pots and pans overflowing in the kitchen sink.

While there, Michelle and I did our best to clean up around the apartment, but we probably spent a good hour in the kitchen alone.

Vincent had grown a ponytail that was in a rubber band at the top of his head and probably went down to his waistline; I'd never seen a six-year-old boy with a ponytail. Vincent loved it, and Debbie let him keep it. For that matter, she pretty much let him do what he wished; she unfortunately had no choice.

My thoughts were interrupted when Vincent momentarily stopped playing his game, looked up at me, and said, "You're Uncle Mike, silly."

Yep, I'm silly Uncle Mike, I thought. I laughed out loud. I asked him what he had been up to lately, and he suddenly got really excited and proceeded to tell me about a sleepover that he had with his friend from the apartment downstairs, but not before making two trips to the bathroom. I smiled and reached over and hugged him; I told him how much I loved him, and he reciprocated. My eyes welled up with tears as we stared at each other for what seemed like an eternity. As with all my family, my love was real. I then got up and made my way into Debbie's bedroom. I felt nervous.

I could feel the nighttime coolness of the October winds rattling their way through the single-pane glass of the windows as soon as I walked over the bedroom threshold. I went around the room and closed the heavy drapes and turned up the heat as there was a definite chill in the room, and I knew that my sister already didn't feel well; she did not need to catch a cold.

I'm not sure what happened to me or what came over me; all I can say is that while she was talking, I didn't hear a single word. I was daydreaming about the condition that she was in, and I pitied her; I wanted to take her away from here. The phone rang, interrupting our one-way conversation. It was a friend of the family who had been looking after Debbie and Vincent. Michelle answered the phone and went into the other room to talk with her; either the conversation was not meant for our ears or she was simply being polite, but I believed it to be the former.

As Debbie lay there, partly propped up by a stack of pillows, she asked how I liked her new apartment and the decorating that she did in the room. We started laughing.

"Michael, Peggy wants to talk to you. Do you have a moment?"

"Sure, I'll talk to her; give me just a minute."

"Sorry, Debbie, yeah, I really like your new place, and your room is absolutely huge." Debbie was always looking for affirmation from me. I never understood why. "The decorating suits you well. Are you still cold?" I asked.

"Yeah, kind of. Would you mind grabbing some blankets out of the chest at the end of the bed?"

I got up from the bed and grabbed a couple of heavier blankets from the cedar chest. I loved the smell of cedar and buried my face into the blankets. I neatly unfolded them and covered her with them. I rearranged her pillows and propped her up higher in her bed. "Are you comfortable now?" I asked.

"Yeah, that feels much better, but I'm worried about the heating bill. I won't be able to afford it if you keep it turned up," she said.

"Your health is more important than a heating bill; send me the bill if you can't afford it," I said. It was evident by the pile of toys on the other side of the bed that Vincent most likely spent his nights with his mother. Vincent was Debbie's entire world. She revolved around him like the earth around the sun, each benefiting from the other's gravitational pull. The love they had for each other was indivisible.

Michelle walked in and handed me the phone. Peggy was an old friend of the family, and she and Debbie had once again ignited a friendship that, for whatever reason, had been allowed to die out a while back. "Hi, Peggy, how are you doing? It's great to hear from you," I said.

"Oh, I'm doing fine. The question is really how are you doing, Michael?" I handed the phone back over to my wife and buried my face in my hands. I instantly burst out crying hysterically. What had come over me? I was supposed to be the strong one.

Debbie sat upright and hugged me tightly.

"Don't cry, Michael. It's OK; I'm OK," she said.

I apologized to her for that was the only thing that I could do. I asked her to lie back down, and I covered her back up once again. I told her I was OK, that my outburst was completely unexpected, and that I was just happy to finally see her again. I gave her a gentle kiss on her cheek and warmed her face with my hands.

I overheard Peggy ask Michelle if I was OK. Michelle told her that I was but that the situation could be a little overwhelming at times. She always seemed able to keep her composure during the tough times, of which we had plenty. This entire situation was simply wrong, but there was nothing that I could do about it. I felt horrible; I felt sad; I felt grief.

LIFE AND DEATH

On a long enough timeline, time may very well heal all wounds. Not true of my sister, however. For my sister, no amount of time or therapy would help heal the wounds associated with adoption. I can't say for sure what it that bothered her so much about finding out this information so many years ago, especially from such a loving and caring person as my mother. Maybe it was her physical age; maybe it was her mental age. Some of us have the ability to move on with life regardless of how devastating circumstances may be; for others, the ability to move on seems to come equipped with a broken stoplight that never changes from red. My sister seemed unable to accept my parents for who they were. There were three things in particular that she did as she grew older just to spite my parents, and they were bad enough that she never told me.

I was at work on May 11, 2000, doing what I always do. There was nothing out of the ordinary, no inkling or foresight that something was catastrophically wrong with the universe that day. Should there have been? Should some messenger perhaps be sent to notify you when your world is about to be turned upside down? Maybe in a universe so complex, so mysterious, someone is whispering to us; it would be a tragedy if he or she was, and we were too busy answering the work phone to pay attention.

I received a call from my mother that afternoon. She quietly asked if it would be possible for me to drive back home that day. Why the whispering? I wondered. Who was being disturbed, my mother or me? My hands went numb as if they were falling asleep. For a moment I thought I might drop the receiver onto my desktop, which would've made a real racket. Instinctively, I lowered my voice to match that of my mother. I did not wish my colleagues to hear my conversation. "You want me to drive home today, Mom?" I asked.

Again the whispering. "I was wondering if it would be possible for you to leave work early and drive home right now."

I felt like I had fallen asleep at the wheel at sixty miles an hour and had run a red light, plowing directly into a family of five driving their minivan on the way home from a birthday party. My forehead began to sweat, and my heart began to pound. This was not news of the obvious kind; something horrible had happened, and I was 350 miles away from where I needed to be in order to have any effect on the situation.

As I could find no words to answer my mother's simple question, I heard her call to me again on the other end of the receiver. "Michael, did you hear me? Can you come home, please?"

Please? Who was I that my mother thought she needed to say please? "Mom, I'm over three hundred and fifty miles away from home and even traveling at the fastest, safest speed, it will still take me close to five hours to get home," I said. I needed to know. I had to ask the one question that I knew no matter what would cause my body to turn to gelatin. "Mom, please tell me what's wrong. What happened?"

"It's your sister…"

I hung up the receiver and phoned Michelle on the way home. I told her there was something wrong with my sister and that my mother had just called me, begging me to come straight home.

As I drove home to gather some clothes and meet Michelle, I suddenly found it strange that she had asked no questions. She never even said anything about her work or the possibility of not being able to go. Had I just missed it, or did she know something I did not?

Michelle was already home by the time I pulled into the driveway. The garage door was open, and two suitcases sat inside. My mobile phone rang as I pulled up, and Michelle indicated that she would be out shortly. Those suitcases had been prepacked; they were not thrown together in any hurry. She knew more than I for the moment. As I backed down the driveway, I asked her if she would mind telling me what was going on as my mother was acting strange enough, not to mention that I was about to break every speed limit in the state in order to get back to St. Louis.

She sat quietly before speaking, and then said that she thought it would be better to talk about it once we got on the highway. I phoned my mother from the car and told her that we were on the way. She thanked me, which I couldn't help but think was odd.

Highway 55 southbound, with cruise control set at eighty miles per hour, I asked Michelle to please tell me what was going on with my sister.

"Your sister has been living in hospice for some time now, and she is dying of melanoma."

I barely missed the highway divider as I swerved the wheel across two lanes of traffic and up the off-ramp. I heard the blare of horns fading in the background and could only pray that I had not caused any accidents. I swerved right, yielding into traffic so as to avoid any lights and hung another hard right into the first gas station in my path, slamming on my brakes. Hot coffee was strewn across my dash, and a fine mist of it quickly permeated the car as it dripped down in front of the air vents.

"What the hell did you just do that for? You could have seriously injured someone!" she said.

"Why the hell didn't you tell me what was going on with my sister, for Christ's sake?" I asked.

"Michael, you knew she had melanoma; certainly you knew this time had to come," she said.

"No, Michelle, I didn't because no one told me what was going on. No one told me things had come to this point. She had melanoma, and I knew that she was sick, but I also knew that she was getting treatment at Barnes-Jewish. Jesus, I've been living a lie. I thought the treatments were going well. What the hell happened? Why did no one say anything to me?" I asked.

"We have, Michael. I'm sorry; I don't know what to tell you. Please, don't be mad at us, but we had been keeping you informed. Your sister, at some point, told the doctors that if there were no further improvements with the medications that she was taking that she was done with them altogether," Michelle said.

Suddenly I remembered; I remembered her threatening to give up. But I knew my sister; I knew her to be incapable of quitting, especially when she had the love of her life to look after, her six-year-old son, Vincent Daniel Seliner, who she had told no one about until she was six months pregnant. There were two things that she stole from my mother and father—the knowledge of having and preparing for a grandson and the knowledge of having and preparing for a dying daughter. Shortly before her death, she even had the gall to get married just for the sake of changing her family name.

"Michael, I don't know exactly what's going on right now with Debbie. You know as well as I that she gave up on life almost a year ago, and she has apparently decided to pull the plug all for the sake of not allowing your parents ample time to prepare for a proper funeral. I'm sorry if you don't recognize this fact, but that's really what's going on here. I only received the same phone call that you did while at work. Why don't you call your mother right now and talk with her? Find out for sure, Michael," she said.

"No, I can't afford to lose the time. Let's just get going. I'm sorry," I said. "This is all part of her master plan to cause turmoil in our family and turn family members against one another. I, for one, won't let that happen."

At twilight, we arrived at the hospice facility where Debra was staying in Southeast Missouri. There were but a handful of cars remaining in the parking lot and not a person in sight. Michelle gently grabbed my arm from the steering wheel. I don't know how long I had been sitting there with my teeth clenched, my tongue pressed tightly up against the roof of my mouth, and my knuckles white from grasping the steering wheel for the past five hours. I was trying desperately to prepare myself for what I thought I was about to see.

"Michael, your parents are in there waiting for us. Go be with your sister, and I'll be there if you want me," Michelle said. What I had secretly wished for was for no one besides my mother and I to be inside with Debbie.

I knew that I couldn't tolerate my dad's aggravation, his nervousness, his constant fidgeting. I would have told him to have a cigarette if I didn't know that he would completely relapse. My wish was selfish and was not to be granted. I walked inside the building that housed the dying, holding hands with my wife, and met my parents at the receptionist's desk.

My mother had been crying; her eyes were red and swollen. She searched in her purse to find more tissues. She hugged me and began to cry uncontrollably. For the first time that I could remember in a long time, my mother cried; she cried for the impending loss of a daughter. It was a loss that I could not even begin to comprehend.

I quietly asked her what exactly the problem was and where Debbie was.

Battling through the tears, she managed to utter the words that Debbie was dying and that we had arrived just in time to say good-bye. She pointed down the hall-way with a shaky hand and indicated that she was in the first room on the right.

I asked if Debbie wanted to see me alone or if she wanted my mother to come back. Crying heavily again, my mother grabbed my arm and walked me down the hallway toward my sister's room. I tried to calm my mother to the best of my abilities. It was a moment in time that I did not want to be. I looked back at Michelle and shook my head for her to remain by the receptionist.

I went into the room and saw my sister curled up into a fetal position, her mouth hanging partly open, staring straight ahead. I had no idea whether she recognized me or even knew that anyone else had entered the room. I immediately broke down and cried uncontrollably. I turned around and quickly walked back out the door as I did not wish for my sister to notice me crying; I had to be the strong one.

My mother scurried out of the room and into the large, open hallway, trying to catch up with me, gently calling repeatedly for me to stop. I couldn't stop. I needed a place to be alone, a place to recompose myself. I headed out the side door of the facility and found my father and wife sitting at the table talking. The crashing open of the double doors must have startled them both as they quickly stood up, their faces filled with fear. This was the last place that I wanted to be as I knew my mother would soon follow.

I was upset and angry, but I was confused most of all. I simply could not put the pieces of this life-and-death puzzle together. There were missing pieces strewn about, and I had no idea where they lay. I could not get over the idea that, had I known, I would have been able to help my sister sooner. My guard was down; I did not expect to be walking into that situation. I felt as though I had been stabbed in the back.

I didn't speak a word; I didn't have to as the expression on my face said everything. My mother tried to comfort me; I would have expected nothing less. I could not be mad at her; no, I knew the fault lay with me. I was to blame for literally not paying attention, not wanting to pay attention. The side door opened once again, and I thought for a moment that it was a nurse coming out to grab a smoke, but instead she indicated that Debbie wanted to see me. I quickly followed the nurse back into the building; there was no time to regain my composure.

I went into my sister's room, grabbing a white plastic chair along the way, and pulled it right up alongside her. I was scared, but I didn't want her to see that. I had never been in the same room with death before. I cursed its name; why now, you bastard? I was upset and wanted to cry, but I didn't want her to see that. I whispered softly to my sister. I had no idea what was registering in her mind; I didn't even know if she could hear me, but at that moment, I didn't care.

"Debbie, it's your brother, and I'm here now," I said. I held her ice-cold hands in my mine. I felt the warmth from my own hands radiating to hers. She was cold, and I noticed a slight shiver come over her. My mother asked the nurse for some warm blankets. Dammit, I was pissed off! How could my sister be lying there in that condition? How could anyone else have not noticed how cold and trembling she was? I wanted to grab a doctor, a nurse, someone, and just literally start beating the hell out of him or her.

Debbie's lips began to move slowly; she was trying to speak but could not be heard. I turned my head to the side, where my ear could pick up the almost indistinguishable words that she spoke next. "Michael, please promise me that you will take care of Vincent forever…" she said.

I knew exactly what she wanted, and while I had no idea what my parents' plans were, I already knew what mine were. I whispered back into her ear, "Debbie, I love you very much, more than you probably ever knew, and I promise you that I will always be there for Vincent. I promise you that I will make him part of my family."

She slowly closed her eyes and drifted off to sleep; she would not awake, not even by the kiss of a prince.

My loving sister, Debra, passed away on May 11, 2000, from melanoma. She died at a tender age of twenty-nine years; I was thirty-two. We were brother and sister, both still children. I felt obligated, compelled, to deliver her eulogy to a gathering of a couple hundred that came together to celebrate her life.

To My Loving Sister, Debra.

Today, I stand here before you all,
nervously looking for the words
to describe her, standing tall,
the sister whom I lost in life
but search for with all my measures.

I can only say I love you,
and thank you for all the treasures.
I wished to deliver this eulogy to you
for the sake of others, including
your only son, Vincent Daniel Seliner,
so they too may know the sister who I grew up
loving so much.

Standing before this loving
gathering on this beautiful morning,
I realize that I was not the only one
whose life you had come to touch so boldly.

I realize only because you taught me
that it's not always the similarities that hold the key
to bringing us together, but the differences
inherent in all of us needed to agree.
I knew and loved you for who
you were born to be,
not for who I wished you to be;
now I can clearly see.

You fought a fight that even the strongest
among us would be proud to say

that they accomplished, that
they fought every day.
In death, there is no failure, no judgment made
by those who love you, whose hearts still ache.
Your life will never fade.

Debra, your prophecy came true,
that you were placed on this earth
to raise an only son, to give birth.
You left us too early
to complete your only task,
but not to worry, all you had to do was ask.

You may rest in peace now;
it's time to move on.
You have done your job; you
have done your part.
It is my turn now, my turn to
step up and have the heart.
As your big brother, I will walk with your son
the rest of the way to manhood.
I will become his father, like
any good man should.

—Always and forever,
Michael

CELEBRATIONS

May 24, 2000.

oward the end of the month, my wife and I made our way back up to Chicago, but this time we were caring a little extra luggage by the name of Vincent Daniel, my adopted nephew. After a short legal-custody battle with Vincent's biological father, we moved forward with adoption and planned out the beginning of the rest of six-year-old Vincent Daniel's life.

I found it odd that even for a six-year-old boy, death did not register as part of the reality that he painted with his little fingers. In the pictures that he painted, there were two mommies and now one Uncle Mike—a father at least from my hopeful viewpoint. Sometimes we asked who the people were in the pictures he painted, but we rarely got a coherent answer, maybe a giggle, maybe a shrug of the shoulders, maybe a finger pointing at one of us. It was clear to us then that death was not just a foreign concept that would be hard for Vincent to reconcile with as a six-year-old; it simply didn't exist. His innocence tugged at my heart. In many respects, we were working with a clean slate; there were no prereconciled conditions.

Debra had done an excellent job raising this young boy from an infant to a six-year-old with what little she had. As we drove back home down the highway, his imagination ran wild, and he began to become more boisterous in his actions and commentary. This was his first trip out of the state, and it showed. He seemed amazed by the simple things that he saw along the highway that we all take for granted: tractors, farm equipment, cows, and even horses—all things of ordinary life that had previously been nothing more than plastic toys in this boy's imagination. His excitement was contagious. I laughed out loud when I heard him scream in excitement over these mundane creatures that had magically come to life.

Michelle and I had decided beforehand that the discussion of his mother's death would wait until sometime after we got home. Debra had made the decision to be cremated, so there was no closure to be found in witnessing the body of his mother. Given the option, I can't really say for certain that I would want a six-year-old seeing the dead body of his mother in a casket.

We had made plans to stop at a McDonald's for dinner on the way home. Although I wasn't hungry, I sat with my wife, drinking a Diet Coke and watching my nephew play for an hour straight within the confines of the indoor jungle gym until we had to pull the plug out of the drain. He reminded me of a chimpanzee at a zoo, and he made all the sound effects to go along with his newfound persona. We got home around seven that evening to the condominium that my work had put me up in until I found a new home following our move from Denver in 1999. I knew it would be hard on Vincent, having to move twice in as many months, but we had no choice; it simply was our reality.

It was my job to put Vincent down for sleep, and Michelle took care of the unpacking from our short but draining trip. I believe that Vincent thought he was spending some time with his aunt and uncle as he was more than happy to see us and wanted to explore the two-story condominium.

I promised him that he could watch TV with me for approximately thirty minutes if promised to go straight to bed afterward. At the time, I enjoyed watching *The X-Files*, which was a sci-fi featured hit on Fox. Personally, I don't think it would've made a difference what I wanted to watch; he would have sat almost on top of me, watching the same program. Surprisingly, he was extremely quiet and said little while the program was on. At times I had to look down at his face to see if he was still awake, and to my surprise, he was intently watching the show. He simply spread out on the couch with his head on my lap. I gently scratched his head to his delight. I gave him an extra fifteen minutes before taking him into his room, tucking him in, and reading one book of his selection. I don't recall what the book title was, but it took no more than five to ten minutes to read it. He asked me to read it again, but I instead made a bargain with him that I would read one more book of my choosing, to which he quickly agreed.

This time the book was a little longer and for a special reason. I looked down at him when I was halfway through and found him sound asleep. I turned off the bedside lamp and stood for a minute in the doorway taking it all in. I'd just inherited the most precious thing that someone could ask for. I stared at him intently, wondering how I would come to explain to him that his mother had passed away of cancer. How would a six-year-old boy come to reconcile the death of his mother? It was a question that continued replaying in my head on a continuous loop. I was a thirty-two-year-old man who didn't have the answers that he so desperately needed; I'm not sure who did.

I needed some time to my own before I headed upstairs to my wife. I knew she knew this, and I knew that she would be waiting up for me in bed. I grabbed a couple of beers out of the refrigerator and turned the television back on, turning down the volume to a bare whisper. I had not even cracked the top of one of the beer bottles open yet when I started sobbing uncontrollably. "You can't leave, Debbie; you can't leave me alone," I whispered to myself. The past couple weeks had been tough on everyone, but especially on me. They say everyone has skeletons in their closets, and there were only two people who knew what my skeletons were—my wife and God. I felt ashamed now, ashamed that I had not been there for my sister earlier when she needed me the most. I cried like a baby, and my God, the relief from that cry felt better than any I had ever had before.

The dam had opened and the emotions poured out. I knew that Michelle could hear me crying loudly, and she came down with the comforter and a couple of pillows, knowing that we would feel better beneath them, just the two of us holding each other tightly. We had each other to look after now, and we were starting to look more like a real family. We were already expecting our first biological son, Nathaniel Michael Seliner, around the middle of September 2000. It somehow felt good knowing that my firstborn would already have an older brother who would be looking after him.

Michelle approached me, kissed me gently, and lay down by my side. She pulled the comforter up over the both of us. She put the side of her face down on to my chest perhaps, listening solemnly to the beat of my heart. I ran my fingers through her long hair and thought about all of the changes that we had already been through, how some of them didn't seem fair, while others were more than joyous. It was hard for me to get the thought of my sister and my nephew out of my head, but caressing my wife's warm, pregnant stomach and feeling the gentle kicks of our son-to-be awakened life in me once again. I knew then that death would not win. As bad as things sounded or seemed at the moment, joyous life itself would triumph, and it was up to me, my wife, and my God to ensure that was so.

While I lay there with her, I wondered what she was thinking. I knew that we needed to have a discussion about Vincent Daniel. I could sense on some level that she felt cheated by the fact that the family that we had planned together had already started on its own. I had a simple answer for that though, and that answer was

God—God had made the choice for us, and we should both be thankful for that.

I grew up believing that we were never to question God's will and what he had in store for us. Life and all that it brought with it would unfold for each of us like the blossom of a rose. We both knew in our hearts that we could provide a good life for him, for all of our children. As hard as I tried to hold it back, I began sobbing like a child again. I thought of my new son's life, quickly growing within my wife. I did not think about the odds of Nathaniel developing MS later in life; God had a plan for him too. I only thought about the immense love for him that I already possessed.

We were also in the process of having a brand-new house constructed in the suburbs of Chicago, which was fun but extremely draining. It seemed like every day brought with it a new set of deadlines for which we had to make decisions regarding the final build of our home. We were both looking forward to leaving the cramped quarters of our condominium and moving into our thirty-five-hundred-square-foot home. Life may have been hectic and upsetting, but it was also good—we had each other.

When my son, Nathaniel Michael, was born on September 12, 2000, at 11:58 p.m. and the nurse handed him to me, I stared into his bright-blue eyes. He stared back at me intently, and my emotions were overwhelming. On some level, it seemed like he already knew who I was. He had heard my voice while inside my wife's womb. Everything that I've ever experienced was toppled by this one intense feeling of love, protection, and fatherhood that was beyond every expectation I had. Suddenly, my singular lifetime goal of being a loving and protective father became clear. Only God could give one such a gift. It can't be expressed in words; it's something that must be experienced. For the first time since my diagnosis, I was blessed to be able to completely forget about my disease. I was able to walk with my son cradled in my arms. God had answered my prayers and allowed me to walk freely once again. For that moment, I will be forever grateful. I will never forget it.

December 24, 2003.

It was our typical Christmas Eve party with the entire family: brothers, sisters, aunts, uncles, cousins, and friends; there had to have been at least fifty of us. The family and friends on my wife's side of the family was nothing short of astounding; it always amazed me. We normally held these parties at the clubhouses within various family neighborhoods. We tried to mix it up every year so that the scenery didn't get too boring. We always played games after eating a huge buffet-style meal where everybody brought a dish and drank our fair share of alcohol.

There was one game in particular that was actually fun and not corny like most of the others. This was a game of chance, a roll of the dice, a game befitting me. There was always a multitude of presents under the Christmas tree, and each present had a number marked on it. The quantity of gifts dictated the number of dice that would be needed. The basic point of the game was quite simple. All you had to do was to roll the dice, and whatever number you rolled dictated the corresponding present you received. There was a fun twist to the game, however, in that once all of the presents under the tree were exhausted and everyone had at least one gift, we had what was called a trading, or, as I liked to call it, a stealing round. Each person received one roll of the dice, and if he or she so chose, the person could either trade with the person whose gift number corresponded with the roll or keep the gift and pass the dice to the next person. Inevitably, the children always stole the largest gifts thinking that they were getting something special, but a lot of the time people simply put small gifts within large boxes to fool people.

Once we completed the game, it was time to open our presents. I chose to keep my present from the beginning and not trade with anyone.

I was sitting with my parents and my wife and sons together at the same table. I opened my gift, which was rather small, probably about six inches long by four inches tall. I had kind of imagined it as a picture frame from the beginning. On opening it, I was correct in that it was a picture frame; however, there were three pictures within the frame, and they turned out to be ultrasound pictures of our third edition to the family, Grace Jane Seliner, who would be born sometime around mid-May.

Michelle and I had been trying very hard to get pregnant, and during our last effort, I was never notified by the doctor as to whether or not any of the eggs turned out to be viable. Michelle had wanted to keep it a secret. I was completely caught off guard and so ecstatic that I yelled from my chair and held up the picture for everyone to see, saying, "My wife and I are pregnant; my wife and I are pregnant!" Michelle and I hugged, and we both began crying tears of joy for once. Not since Nathan's birth had I felt this way.

September 12, 2008.

Tonight, typing, I can still feel this connection of love as strong as ever. I watch him now, elated by his eighth birthday party. I see his confidence, his strength, and his unwavering love for a father who feels like a failure. Where did the past eight years go? I close my eyes, trying to remember, trying to grasp at the memories of the past eight years. I sit in my wheelchair, bound; my thoughts are lucid, and my love for my kids is as deep as I now realize my parents' was for us.

I am a dad, I should be playing ball with my son, or riding a bike with him, or having a tea party with my four-year-old daughter, Grace Jane. These are the images that society portrays for me. The kids find it fun to push the wheelchair, at least until the typical childhood boredom sets in. I've spent countless hours crying in self-pity, crying in the dark, by myself where no one can see or hear. There have been times when my emotional state has been so low that thoughts of suicide cloud my mind. And then I remember, I remember my children who just don't seem to give a damn that Dad uses a wheelchair to get around. Instead they ask me if I need help or go get help when I truly need it.

Kids are resilient, or so I've been told. "All they need to know is that you love them," I've also been told. Love them? I love them with every fiber of my being. I feel like a towel that has been rung dry. I would give my life to save theirs in a heartbeat. I care about nothing else but taking care of them and giving them all that life has to offer. I am afraid, however, that even knowing all this, I will one day want to find a way out, and it is a feeling that can be so overwhelming that I cannot control it. It is a decision that lies at my very foundation; it is not to be taken lightly.

My eyelids are heavy, and my need for sleep is overwhelming. Suicide is a very dark place; I can only wipe away the tears that have run down my face. My guard is down, my armor is off, I am defenseless, I am not the tough teenager that I once was, and I couldn't care less. I have not been an absentee father; I will not accept that answer. I will not accept death. I must celebrate life; the life that I have with my family. I have been and always will be there for them. I will not quit.

To My Children,
My Heart Beats with Yours

All my life, I've prayed for one thing,
for children to call my own;
my prayers have finally been answered;
my heart no longer beats alone.

The days you were born,
my heart began to beat with yours;
One beat, two beats, three beats, four…
all beats synchronized now with the
conductor's score.

All I ever wanted was for my dreams and choices
to fill a loving house with children's voices.
I close my eyes and I can still hear their laughter,
something for me that has been long sought after.

With hands lifted up to the heavens in prayer,
I pray to God that they're still there.
I pray that not a moment did I waste
as I made a mad dash toward
that finish line in haste.

Never taking the time to watch what I should
but instead only hearing what I could.
I shed a tear for them now,
maybe a moment too late
as I missed every run across home plate.

I hope that one day they will understand.
I pray that one day they will take a stand,

one that they can call their own,
and not march to the beat of another drone.

—Love, Dad

Chipping Away the Stone

June 8, 2007.

"It's been a few months since I've seen you last, Mike. How have you been feeling?" Bob asked.

"Do you know that when Michelangelo was asked how he made it look so easy to sculpt the human form, he said, 'Sculpting is easy; you just go down to the skin and stop'?" I said. "I find it so amazing how great thinkers and inventors all have at least two things in common. First, they all think outside the box, and, second, none of them are afraid of failure. Even Michelangelo has been quoted as saying, 'Faith in oneself is the best and safest course.'"

"It sounds like you've been doing some pretty deep thinking since we've talked last. What's the reason for this?" Bob asked.

"I'm not certain, but maybe it just comes with all of the crap that I have been through as of late. I'm trying to place myself outside of that box to help solve my problems in a different manner because what I am doing now is not working. Hopefully, placing myself outside of the box will help me reconcile with my problems. This is my life, and it's ending one minute at a time. It just seems to me that every time things start off well, they take a divergent path and leave me empty-handed," I said. "I know exactly what Michelangelo is talking about, and it makes perfect sense to me. The question is how to relate what he did to what I am going through."

"Well, Mike, it sounds to me like you have a game plan going forward. Perhaps I can help you chip away some of the stone," Bob said with a grin.

"That certainly would be nice for a change; I mean to actually complete something that I started," I said. "We're still talking about my mental health, aren't we?"

"Of course. Why don't we talk about what you've been up to since we talked last?" Bob asked.

"I've actually been quite busy with various projects. Is there something in particular that you'd like to discuss?" I asked.

"Why don't you pick a subject?" Bob asked.

"OK, well, for starters, I'm leaving Chicago and moving back to St. Louis," I said.

"What? When and how did this come about?" Bob asked, shocked.

"Honestly, I'm sick of my current job. It fucking sucks, and I'm tired of fighting my wife about it," I said.

Bob asked, "Did you quit? Did you already find another job?"

"I can tell that you seemed pretty surprised and maybe a little upset? I guess I shouldn't have sprung this one on you like that. Sorry," I said.

Bob responded, "No, that's quite all right, Mike. That's why we're here, to talk about things like this, right?"

"OK, well, to answer your first question, I guess you could say that I did quit my current job, but I will be staying with the same company, and I'm being transferred to a new division at our St. Louis headquarters. With the transfer, I'll also be moving over to our main engineering branch, which is something I've always wanted. The more I thought about it, the more I agreed that with my disease progressing, we needed more help as a family, and that was only going to happen if we made the move back to St. Louis."

"This sounds like a huge step forward for you, Mike. I have to tell you, I'm really proud of you. One year ago, I would've never expected something like this from you. Congratulations," Bob said with sincerity.

"Thank you, Bob. I appreciate it," I said.

"So tell me what your wife thinks about this move."

"She's absolutely hysterical. I think the day I told her, she actually spent that whole evening on the phone talking with everybody about it. Come to think of it, I know she did because I remember going to bed by myself," I said.

"How much of an influence was she in making the move?" Bob asked.

"She bugged me about it quite a bit, but overall I would say it was fifty-fifty," I said. Well, there you have it, fifty-fifty, another perfect game of coin toss!

"What about your parents? What do they think about it?" Bob asked.

"Oh, they're happier than pigs in slop. My mother has missed seeing the kids so much. I know it had to break her heart, but we won't have to worry about that anymore, will we?" I said.

"I have a question to ask," I said. "I never thought I'd be admitting this, but I think that I'm probably going to need at least one, if not more, sessions with you before I feel totally comfortable walking away."

Bob responded by saying, "Yeah, I figured we'd get around to that sooner or later; sooner's fine. What did you have in mind?"

"Well, I wondered if you would be open to having a phone session. I'd like to set it up for two hours, and I'd make it worth your while since the insurance company probably won't cover it," I said.

"Yeah, that sounds like a good idea, and I'm sure we can work something out from the payment stand-point—don't worry about that," Bob said.

"Great, I'm glad to have that off my chest," I said.

"Wow, you're making a lot of progress right off the bat here. Do you have more good news for me?" Bob asked.

"If I can think of some, Bob, you'll be the first to know, OK?" I said. "I'd like to talk to you about my marriage."

"Oh, that doesn't sound too good. What's going on?" Bob asked.

"Well, I guess I have what you would call a two-part problem, and for the life of me, I don't know how to solve part one," I said.

"Go on; I'm listening," Bob said.

"OK, both parts have to do with the sexual part of our relationship. I'm sure you're aware with what you've read about MS that sexual dysfunction can be a typical problem. Well, it just so happens that for me it is a prob-lem, a big one," I said.

"Are you on an ED medication?" Bob asked.

"Yeah, I'm on Viagra, and I have so much of it that I could distribute it on the streets if I wanted to, but that's not the issue," I said.

"Is the Viagra not working?" Bob asked.

"It's a tough question for me to answer; sometimes it does help me out, and other times, it doesn't do anything. I really have no way of predicting when it may work or not, and it's pretty disturbing to me, actually embarrassing," I said.

"Have you talked to your PCP about it?" Bob asked.

"Yeah, I have, and he's had me try the other drugs, all of which have the same effect. After talking with him about it for a while, he suggested that the problem may be more related to MS than anything else and that no drug or no amount of drugs may work," I said.

"How have you been dealing with the issue then, Mike? Maybe I should ask how you and Michelle are dealing with the issue," Bob asked.

"Well, this is where the issue kind of blends into part two, which is me not really wanting to or, I should say, feeling like having sex in the first place," I said.

"Well, Mike, there're a few questions that I have stemming from that statement. First off, I have to ask you if you feel that you are really still in love with your wife? How long has it been since you guys have had sexual relations?" Bob asked.

I knew that if I was to truly get any help whatsoever, I had to be completely honest with the one person I trusted at this point. It was a difficult question to answer. I responded by saying, "Bob, I'm in love with my wife today as much as the day that we got married; nothing has changed. The problem truly lies in the fact that I feel like I have no libido. In other words, I simply have no desire to be with my wife sexually, and I find it very aggravating knowing how much she wants to be with me."

"OK, well, if that is the case, then I think that your PCP may be correct in stating that the problem may stem from MS itself, and if so, it's completely out of your control," Bob said. "Have you talked with your wife about this issue and what your PCP has said?"

"No, I simply can't find the courage to tell her that I have no desire to be with her sexually but that I still love her more than ever," I said. "A conversation like that would not go over too well because she has already made inferences to the fact that she could not live in a loveless relationship."

"It may sound silly, but do you feel that you are you using sex as a weapon? In other words, are you withholding sex from her because you may be angry with her or something along those lines? Bob asked.

"No, that's absolutely ridiculous. I love my wife, and when we do have arguments, we normally work them out and move on. It's always been an agreement that we've had for a long time—we don't let issues lie, and we never go to bed angry. I've never withheld sex from her for any reason," I said.

"What does Michelle have to say when this happens?" Bob asked.

"Well, I've got it tell you that it's pretty fucking embarrassing for a man not to be able to get an erection and have sex with his wife. She gets pretty upset, and I would say even angry over it as she thinks that I simply don't want to have sex with her, which as I said before is simply not true," I said.

"You realize, Mike, that sometimes even for married couples there's a lot of pressure to perform, especially in scenarios such as yours. Do you understand that? Do you talk to her about your problem?" Bob asked.

"Good question. What am I supposed to say to her? Oh, well, better luck next time? Like I said, she gets really upset, which ends up putting a lot of pressure on me and makes me angry and defensive in turn. Because of that, I avoid talking to her about it. It's a vicious cycle, and I'm just sick of it," I said.

"Mike, have you ever even had one single constructive conversation with her about this matter?" Bob asked.

"Honestly, no, not one," I said.

"For the sake of your marriage, don't you think that she deserves to hear the truth? I'm just saying she could be totally understanding of your situation, which would take the pressure off of you. You never know, it may be the pressure itself that is causing you a mental block of sorts from actually getting an erection, especially if the doctor is telling you that there's nothing wrong with you physically. Besides, there are other things that you can do together as a couple that may satisfy her," Bob said.

Bob was right, and I should've ended the conversation with him right then and there. I should've marched home and spoken with my wife and told her the truth about what was going on with me, but I didn't. Why?

"Mike, I have one more question for you, and please don't get upset with me—this is just a textbook question, OK?" Bob said.

"OK," I said.

"Do you still have sexual feelings for your wife? In other words, are you still attracted to her, do you still want to be with her sexually?" Bob asked.

"Another good question, Bob. It's complicated because the answer is not a simple yes or no in my mind. I would have to say that I really don't have any sexual feelings for her anymore," I said.

"So to be clear, you don't even really want to be with her from the sexual standpoint, is that correct?" Bob asked.

"I would say that's correct, but I also have to tell you that I still love her very, very much, and I really do want to be with her, just on a different level," I said. "Does that make sense?"

"Yes, I think I understand what you're trying to tell me. You still want to be with your wife, just not on the sexual level?" he asked.

"That's exactly right," I said.

I heard Bob's advice, and I know that while it sounds simple, I wouldn't take it. My wife wanted to have sex; she didn't want to snuggle. Hell, before I had MS, we had sex all the time and we snuggled, but the snuggling that always led to the sex. It was a vicious cycle, and I didn't care as long as I was getting what I wanted out of it also. I don't blame her; if the tables were turned, I'd probably feel the same way.

"Bob, I don't know how much longer she's going to stick around with me. I've got to figure something else out before she ends up leaving," I said.

I'm lying completely horizontal in my reclining wheelchair. I'm on my back staring up at the glass ceiling. Bob finally forked out some cash and got those windows tinted. Son of a bitch, I can't believe he actually took my advice. Maybe that's why he didn't ask my permission to turn on the ceiling fan earlier. "Bob, how's the window tinting working out for you?" I asked.

"Oh, yeah, I forgot to mention that to you. I can't believe the difference that it made. The guy who came out gave me a quote and recommended that I go with the five percent grade tint. He said it would make it a lot darker in the room but that it would have the greatest effect on my cooling bill. I haven't had a chance to check my bill yet as I haven't gone through a full quarterly cycle, but I can already tell the difference myself. I haven't had to turn the fan on once since getting the tint installed, so I'm looking forward to seeing how it really performs through the summer. I owe you a big thanks," Bob said.

"No problem; maybe I'll let you take me to Ruth's Chris for a nice steak," I said. "You don't mind me lying down like this, do you? I don't want to seem rude; it's just that talking about a lot of this stuff makes me sleepy, relaxed for some reason."

"Yeah, it feels good to get a lot of this stuff off your chest, doesn't it?" Bob asked. He never bothered asking me if I wanted a cup of hot tea, but I wasn't touching that conversation with a ten-foot pole. I wouldn't even look over there.

From my new vantage point, I had a perfect view of that new cheap-ass clock that he hung from one of the main wooden support columns in his office. It was one of those analog clocks that schools must have purchased by the barge load. Real classic, the second hand was even off by about two degrees in either direction. Every time it clicked off another second, the red second hand jerked past its intended stop point and then moved counterclockwise ever so slightly. He probably hung it up there with a thumbtack. The whole contraption just reeked of cheapness and was kind of the polar opposite of Bob's personality. Strange, but I wasn't going to get into it with him. If he wanted to look cheap, that was his problem, not mine.

"Do you think you want to go ahead and schedule our appointment for next week, Mike, or how do you want to handle this?" Bob asked.

"Well, with everything that I have going on, I think we better wait and let me get my schedule penned in before giving you any dates that you may have to change. Sound fair?" I asked.

"Sounds good to me. You have my number, so give me a call. I just ask that you try your best to give me a week's notice, especially if you want to have a two-hour session, OK?"

"No problem, Bob. Will do. And listen, I really mean it when I say that it's been a real pleasure, and I appreciate all your help to date," I said.

"Same here, Mike, and hopefully I'll be talking to you soon," Bob said.

PROGRESS

July 2, 2007.

The move back to St. Louis was years overdue, at least from my wife's standpoint. Sometimes I feel like I'd still be living in Chicago, stuck in the quagmire, had Michelle not pushed the issue to return back home so much. However, I was glad that my kids finally got to spend some quality time with their grandparents and extended family members; I felt like they were missing out on too much with their family as they grew older.

I have to admit to a little trepidation not just in starting a new job but mainly in having a lot of old friends I had not seen in a while see me in a wheelchair for the first time. I should have talked with Bob about this issue prior to leaving, but I knew that the best way to solve the issue was by simply jumping into the frying pan so to speak. I had an appointment with Bob for the next day, so I would be able to still discuss these things with them prior to heading back to work. My friends were my friends; no one was going to jump ship just because they found me in a wheelchair. The whole point was ludicrous, and I can't believe I let my mind go down that path, but those are some of the thoughts that go through the mind of a handicapped person—worry.

My physical health had been deteriorating in general over the past few months, and I would normally attribute it to the added stress of moving; however, this time, I wasn't sure of the cause. I had been experiencing a lot of spasticity in my lower extremities, which caused me a great deal of pain that was not under control with my current medication of OxyContin.

My move back to St. Louis coincided with my need to replace my ITB (Intrathecal Baclofen) pump. These pumps are typically implanted into the left or right abdomen and have a catheter that delivers medication directly from the pump to the lumbar portion of the spinal column. The ITB medication itself is what ultimately controls and stops the spasticity in the lower extremities (the legs).Most of the pumps are variable speed, allowing the doctor to adjust the amount of medication that is ultimately delivered to the lumbar spinal column. For patients who have maximized their intake of oral Baclofen, the ITB pump is the last viable resort.

The good part about getting an ITB pump, however, is that very little ITB medication is required relative to the oral drug because the medication is delivered directly to the spinal cord. The only real downfalls to the ITB pump are that the patient needs to have the pump refilled in a sterile setting approximately every three months, and the pump itself will need to be surgically replaced every five years. This just happened to be one of those years and, to be more specific, one of those weeks.

July 3, 2007—Moving Day.

We planned the holidays to be a busy time, not just for my family but for everyone involved with our move. The moving truck from Chicago left the past weekend and arrived on July 2 to start unloading the trailer. One would never perceive that all of your belongings from a thirty-five-hundred-square-foot house would fit into one tractor-trailer. It really is amazing how large these machines are; you just don't recognize it while they're on the highway passing you at eighty miles per hour.

While our families planned to help unpack our belongings, I had to prepare for surgery, which was scheduled for eleven that morning. It was to be a minor surgery and would not last for more than thirty minutes. The nice part was that it was outpatient surgery since this was my second pump, so I was now on my tenth year with this type of pump. The difficult part was yet to come, however, as after implantation of the pump began the fine-tuning stage, in which the ITB pump speed was incrementally increased in order to reach a "floating goal." A floating goal is simply a target amount of medication that is required in order to either help you walk better or reduce the amount of spasticity encountered. There is no preset goal or amount of medication plotted on a chart in a doctor's office somewhere. While not completely experimental, it is very close to it. The key is patience, and patience can pay huge dividends.

After only my second day of ITB pump adjustments, I was able to completely eliminate all spasticity from my lower extremities. This was an incredible leap forward given that after my first pump implantation, it took upward of six months to get the pump to where I could actually feel my legs. As a matter of fact, the first pump implantation was such a setback for me that I had considered removing it altogether.

DIVORCE

April 9, 2009.

It was a late afternoon in early spring when Michelle called me at work a couple of hours prior to my leaving. I hadn't noticed the time as I had been lost in my work, but I would say that it was around six—another late night. Once I noticed the time, I realized that she was calling to find out when I planned to come home; dinnertime was usually around six. I was about to tell her that I was going to cut my time short and would be home within a half hour when I noticed an uneasiness about her voice. I asked her if there was a problem and if she needed me home earlier.

"Yes, I would appreciate it if you could come home as soon as possible," she said.

"What's going on, Michelle?" I asked.

"I'd really just prefer to talk about it once you get home, OK?" she replied.

I asked her where the kids were, and she replied that they were over at her parents' house visiting and having dinner. I immediately recognized that something was seriously wrong, as my kids very rarely visited Michelle's parents on their own. "I'll be home in a few minutes, OK?" I said.

"OK," she replied.

I lived approximately twenty miles away from work, so it usually took me about thirty minutes to get to and from work with no traffic. I was already sick to my stomach, that instant uneasiness that you get upon hearing bad news and one that an entire bottle of Tums could do nothing about. Had I had any food in my gut, I would have puked it out. A discussion alone with my wife in a house void of people? I was already thinking the worst, and my right foot became a brick on the car's throttle as I drove home.

I opened the laundry-room door and immediately looked in at the kitchen table to see Michelle sitting there already, alone. Her hands covered her face, and I could tell that she was crying. Somebody died, I thought. I dropped my workbag on the kitchen tile and quickly walked over toward my wife, who, by then, had stood up from the table, backed away from me, and stared at me with a queer look about her face.

I reached out for a hug as I normally did upon returning from work, but there was no reciprocation, only ice-cold silence. "What the hell is going on, Michelle?" I asked. "What's wrong?" Questions to no avail; I couldn't even get her to look at me now as her attention was drawn to the floor.

She stood at the far end of the table, a sweeping rectangular table about three feet by seven feet with the leaf in it.

The kitchen table centerpiece was missing or had been taken away; it was one of Michelle's favorites. What an odd thing to notice, I thought.

"Can you go sit at the other end of the table, please?" she asked.

"Do you have to sit at this end of the table?" I asked.

"Please just have a seat, Michael. There's something I need to talk to you about," she replied. I could tell that she had been crying for some time as her eyes and face were puffy and red. The sides of her hair were wet from her tears. For a moment, the only thing I wanted to do was get back in my car and drive to my parents' house. I had left my phone in my car, and for some reason, I had an uneasy feeling that perhaps my kids were not with Michelle's parents but with someone else.

My anger and anxiety began to boil over again as I felt that I was not being given the answers that I deserved. I called her name, but she interrupted me and proceeded to talk. Finally some answers.

"Michael, I'm leaving you," she said before bursting into tears.

"Like hell you're leaving me. Who the hell do you think you are, and what the hell is really going on here?" I asked.

"Like I said, I've made the decision to leave you, and I'm asking you for a divorce," she said.

"You're asking me for a divorce?" I asked laughingly. My guise of laughter was a thin veil covering a near breakdown. I refused to start crying in front of her, in front of this bitch who had betrayed me at the highest level. "I'm glad you had the time to make a decision to leave me right out of the blue, but I'll tell you right now, there's no chance in hell that I'm simply going to give you a divorce for no reason. What have I done to you, Michelle? What have I said to you, Michelle, that would deserve you divorcing me? I love you, as in still in love with you, and suddenly you throw this shit on me?" I asked. "What am I supposed to do, I mean with myself, Michelle? What the hell am I to do?"

For once, my rage was nothing but that, rage. There was no other meaning behind it. I wanted to strike out, to strike back more precisely. I could think of nothing but how my disease had betrayed me once again. As

I had asked her, what the hell was I supposed to do? Where the hell was I supposed to go? What the hell was going to happen to me?

"Are you seeing someone, Michelle?" I asked. She had left her previous fiancé for me; therefore, I did not put it beyond her to do the same once again to me.

"Michael, there's a lot of stuff that we could go over, but what's the point? I've asked for a divorce, and in the end, I will get a divorce from you. I have obtained an attorney, and I suggest that you do the same as quickly as possible," she said.

"You pompous fucking ass! Who the hell do you think you are?" I asked. "Do you recall your wedding vows? Do you remember the vows that you took in front of Christ Himself on His altar in front of all those witnesses? If you don't, I sure as hell do. Let me repeat them for you. 'Michelle, do you take Michael to be your husband? Do you promise to be true to him in good times and in bad, in sickness and in health, to love him and honor him all the days of your life?' the priest asked. 'I do,' you said.

"Sad, Michelle. This is nothing but sad, and I just don't have any other words for it. I know we've had our problems, but so does every married couple. This is about me having multiple sclerosis, isn't it?" I asked.

"No, Michael, you know that's not true. There's plenty more to this story than you having MS. Please don't try to blame our problems on you having MS," she said.

I replied, "OK, well, if it's more than me having MS, then please, please tell me what are those issues? What is it that's making you want to leave me so suddenly?"

She pulled her hands away from her face again, and while fighting back tears and a bottom lip that would not stop quivering, I could tell that she was starting to become very angry, but at what I didn't know.

"Michael, we live in a loveless relationship. You couldn't care less about being with me or anyone else for that matter. You couldn't care less about being with the kids or even spending time with them. You refuse to go out in public, almost afraid that someone will see you in your walker, denying your kids the simple pleasure of having you around no matter what it is that we may do. These things have nothing to do with having MS. These things have everything to do with living in a loveless relationship," she said.

I drew away from the table, pushing myself off from the end, sliding across the flooring and sitting deeper in the chair well. "This has everything to do with sex and the fact that you're not getting any, am I right? I can't freaking believe you! You know the problems that I have, and you knew about them prior to us getting married. You've got one set of brass balls, and you're talking out both sides of your mouth. You know, I should be the one asking for a divorce from a wife who acts like an absolute child. You think of me not being able to have sex as some sort of joke, and you rub it in my face constantly. You have the nerve to keep a sex calendar, and you mark off each day that you don't get fucked! You think you're the only one living with problems? How many people know about our love life, Michelle? I'll tell you, Michelle—everybody, that's who! Yeah, it's no great mystery what you talk about with your girlfriends; it doesn't take a genius to understand that. I see their glares like I'm some sort of abusive husband. I guess you needed plenty of time to get your cover story straight, huh?" I grabbed my walker with my right hand, picked it off the ground, and threw it up against the island, busting it in half. My rage had reached its peak, and I could tell that Michelle was honestly scared.

I was outraged that she could minimize my disease while talking about its effects in the same sentence. This was typical of Michelle; she had always said and done what she pleased without worrying about the consequences. For her there never were any consequences.

This time, however, was different; this time she had blown the whistle and called an end to our relationship once and for all. She did so with impunity, without my input, without my thoughts, without my feelings. I had no recourse. Her words, her actions, were sharp and quick and cut me deeply and exactly, like a surgeon's knife. There was no coming back from this, I knew that now. I realized that her words had a certain finality to them, and no matter what I said or did, there was no going back. I would fight though; I would fight a useless fight until the end, but what defined the end?

"Two things—first off, I want to know where my kids are, and second, I want you the fuck out of this house right now!" I said. "If you think you're going to continue to live here until I sell this fucking house, you're absolutely crazy."

A certain part of me almost felt relief at the situation at hand. She had said something that struck a nerve of truth in my body. She had said that she was in a "loveless relationship." The truth of the matter was that I really no longer loved her in the sense that she expected. A smirk came across my face, but it was short-lived.

"Michael, what the hell do you find so funny about this situation? Is it something that I said?" she said.

"Yeah, it was everything that you said. It's all simply ludicrous and unbelievable," I said. "You know what,

Michelle, the more I hear you talk, the more it makes me sick. I'm done fucking around with you, and yes, I will get an attorney. I'll give you what you want. I'm so fucking tired of fighting you. I'm just throwing in the towel."

"That's sad, Michael, really sad to hear," she said.

What a coincidence, I thought. Here I was just a short time ago talking to my therapist about my issues with my marriage, all of which have come to fruition over a matter of minutes. Although it made me sick and did no good whatsoever, I finally had the proof that she was highly upset and agitated over the fact that we did not make love according to her schedule of needs, never mind mine. It was too late for talk now, however. All I could do now was to strike back, to do what I knew best. I had taken over my sister's place as the king cobra. I would strike Michelle unsuspectingly and endlessly. I would poison her body with an endless strain of venom for which there was no antitoxin. I would make her suffer one last time. This was my game plan, as ludicrous as it was.

I did not make it into work the following day. I called my boss and told him that I wasn't feeling well. He understood, and no big deal was made out of it.

The truth of the matter was that I was deathly sick. I had thought that my life was over once I heard the diagnosis of

MS, but now that I heard the diagnosis of divorce, I honestly did not know what to do next. I contemplated suicide and thought for hours about what would be the best or easiest method to finally rid myself of all this craziness, of all this nonsense called life. No one deserved to live like that. My mind could take no more; I was running on fumes. I wanted to get in my car and just drive—to where, I know not. My tears were all but dry, and my anger had turned to grief, or, more precisely, loneliness.

I had entrusted my wife with one secret, and now I needed to find another to tell this secret. God, would it ever end? I did not want to confide in anyone at work; things this big had a way of making themselves known to others very quickly, usually without your knowledge. I knew that I had to speak with my mother and try to work out some sort of game plan. I prayed for death. I opened my medicine cabinet and stared at the multitude of medicine bottles. How many and in what combination would it take to make me silently go to sleep forever?

I took a seat on our bathroom floor and stared up at the cabinet for hours, wondering; where was the balance of scales now? I began my departure from reality at that moment; nothing seemed too real any longer. Strange, but a sudden calm came over me in that moment of panic and grief. I knew that Michelle would get what she wanted in the end; would I?

I had called my mother earlier in the morning once Michelle had gone to work and explained to her what had happened the night before. Not surprisingly, she already knew my secret; Michelle had contacted her the day before and had told her what she was planning. God only knows why. Maybe she thought she was protecting me on some level as my mother was planning to come over the following day and would spend some time with me. Honestly, I wasn't sure if I wanted a houseguest, especially during this period of turmoil. Then again, it did make me feel better when I heard that she would be staying. Maybe that's what I needed after all—not silence and loneliness but to be with someone and talk with someone about my problems. One problem that I simply had to try to get over was the fact that I felt my mother had betrayed me on some level by keeping Michelle's secret from me. She had talked for years about all of the issues that she had with Michelle, yet there she was, protecting her.

Later in the morning, not only did I start to feel better, but I decided that going into work and keeping my mind occupied would be better for me than sitting around an empty house. I must have seemed nervous as my colleagues kept asking if I was feeling all right. To me, this was just one more battle that I would have to fight through; there was no backing down. I'm not sure why, but I couldn't stop thinking about my soon-to-be ex-wife sleeping in one of our spare bedrooms. Every time I thought about it, I thought of her being with a different man in my own house, and with it came my old friend rage. I quickly closed the door to my office and dialed her number. Surprisingly, she picked up the phone and told me that she was in a session and would have to call me back when she got out. Before she had the chance to hang up the phone, I quickly told her that I would not allow her back in the house and that she was not to spend the night any longer. I then slammed down the receiver in disgust.

The noise from my office drew attention from my employees. My next phone call was to Michelle's parents to tell them that I was coming over to pick up the kids after work. Our nanny was to pick up the kids from school and drop them off at my in-laws. Call it intuition, I felt something was wrong. I went to grab the receiver when the phone began to ring.

It was my eldest son, Vincent, on the other line, and when I asked him what was going on and if he was OK, he responded by saying, "Well, first off, where are Nathan and Grace? Are they with the nanny? Also, did you know that

I had to walk home from school and that about half of our furniture is gone from the house?"

I felt the heat of rage coming off my face and the palpitations in my pounding heart. I nearly threw the phone through the front glass of my office. "Vincent, are you telling me that your brother and sister are not home and neither is the nanny?" I asked.

"Yep, that's right, Dad. What's going on?" he asked.

Vincent was a freshman in high school now and no longer attended the same school as Nathan and Grace. I realized that he would have no way of knowing where exactly they and the nanny were. Michelle had put together an elaborate plan, one that I did not think she was capable of. Touché.

"Vincent, I need you to do Dad a favor and go into your brother's room while staying on the phone, OK?" I asked. He had to walk up the stairs and go to the other end of the house to get to his brother's room, and I was not looking forward to what my gut told me was about to happen.

"Dad? Are you still there?" he asked. "Yeah, I'm here. Now what I need you to do is go into his drawers and closet, and see if his clothes are still in there, OK?" I asked.

"Dad, all his clothes are gone and so are a bunch of his toys that he had sitting around his room. Did we get robbed or something?" he asked.

"Vincent, I want you to go over to the neighbor's house until I get home, which will be in about thirty minutes, OK? Before you go, can you tell me briefly what furniture is missing from the house?" I asked.

"Like I said before, about half of our stuff is gone. I think that we've been robbed. I'm kind of scared. Can I leave now?" he asked.

"Yeah, Vince, go ahead and get out of the house. Go over to Mary's and call me once you get over there to tell me that you're OK, all right?" I said.

I sat at my desk with the receiver in my left hand up to my ear and my right hand on my forehead with my fingers nervously running through my hair. I couldn't believe that she had already emptied out the house of what I guess she thought were her belongings prior to the divorce. What the fuck was she thinking? I quickly dialed her mother's number again, but no one answered. Caller ID, I thought. There was no way that they were going to pick up the phone, especially not for me. My wife had actually kidnapped my two younger children and had left Vincent to fend for himself and come home to what he saw?

I thought for a minute about why she would have left him to come home to an empty house. It was then that I realized that she left him there because he was not her biological son. Vincent was adopted, and her love for him was different—no, was absolutely lacking. Sad that he would one day understand the full ramifications of this moment that he found himself in. None of the kids needed to be a part of this issue between the two of us. I needed to try to do something.

I called my mother while I was on my way back home and notified her about what was going on. I could tell by her stunned tone that she played no role in this unfolding catastrophe.

"Did you do or say something to her that would make her do what she did, Michael?" she asked.

"No, Mom, that's just it. I've done nothing to deserve to with this level of shit. And what makes me especially sick is the fact that she basically kidnapped our two youngest kids and left Vincent to fend for himself when he came home from school. I should say, after he walked home from school. No one was there to pick him up and take him home. They just left him there at school, Mom. I mean, you should've heard him on the phone. He actually thought that we had been robbed because, according to him, half of our stuff is gone from the house already. And then to think that the nanny played a role in it just makes me wanna swing a golf club upside her noggin. Can you believe all of this?" I asked.

"No, I just can't believe that Michelle would do something like this, especially given your condition and knowing that there's very little that you can do about it. And you're right to say what you did about the nanny. She should have just quit and gone home and stayed out of it altogether, but instead she put herself smack in the middle of a family affair," she said.

"OK, well, I am going to be home in about twenty minutes. Do you think there's any way that you can meet me over there so that I have a witness to what happened? I don't have a camera as I think the batteries are dead, so if you can bring one to take pictures of everything, I would greatly appreciate it," I said.

"OK. I have a really nice digital camera that'll work fine. Are you going to call the police or what?" she asked.

"Yeah, I plan on doing that, but I also need to hire a divorce lawyer as I can see that I'm going to need one," I said.

"OK, I'll see you in about a half hour then," she said.

Once I got home, I called the Jefferson County sheriff's office and explained to them what had happened. They told me that they would send out a sheriff as soon as they had one freed up; apparently they were quite busy dealing with all the Friday afternoon car accidents. My mother

arrived at my home around five thirty and was as astonished as I was about all the property that was missing.

I had called my neighbor Mary on my way home
from work and explained the situation. I asked her if
it would be OK for Vincent to stay at their house for
dinner until I at least got things worked out with the
police. I didn't want Vincent to be a part of any of that
mess.

The Jefferson County sheriff's office sent two squad
cars, which showed up at around six fifteen. One of them
was an unmarked cop in plainclothes, and I assumed
that he was probably a detective. I went over everything
with him from beginning to when Vincent came home
and phoned me at work. The cops didn't seem too bothered by the entire situation, which told me one of two
things: either they had seen this type of shit time and
again, or all of it was completely legal, and they planned
to do nothing.

"Where does your mother-in-law live?" one of the
deputies asked.

"She lives in St. Louis County, over by the new hospital," I said.

"And do you have any idea where your wife may be
right now? Does she or your nanny have a boyfriend
perhaps they may be staying with?" he asked.

I found the question to be rather insensitive, especially given the tone of his voice, which was completely flat and uncaring. He was supposed to be helping me. "Well, I know that my nanny does not have a boyfriend. She has not spoken of even meeting or seeing anyone in the past few years that she's been with us. As for my wife goes, I severely doubt that she does, but I could be wrong. Wherever they are, I know that they're together and that they have the kids. I highly suspect that they are over at my mother-in-law's house right now.

"As far as my furniture, well, that was obviously a planned event in which they were just waiting for me to leave the house so they could come in and take everything. It had to take a small moving company to clear out all of the furniture that I'm talking about. Again, touché on the planning, I thought to myself. Is any of this stuff that we're talking about so far a crime?" I asked.

"Well, it's kind of a tricky situation, and there are some laws governing divorce and who can take what when. To further complicate the matter, the laws are different between Jefferson County and St. Louis County," he said.

"OK, but I obviously live in Jefferson County and the crime, so to speak, was committed here, right?" I asked. *These guys are a bunch of clowns*, I thought.

"You're right, however, as you indicated, you believe that everything that was taken from your house, including your two youngest children, are now within St. Louis County, which is obviously outside of our jurisdiction," he responded.

"So are you saying that I also need to contact St. Louis County police?" I asked.

"I don't think it would be a bad idea, but to be honest with you, it really is going to be quite a mess," he said. "Can I ask you if you've hired a divorce lawyer yet?"

"Yeah, I've hired a local firm, but it won't be official until I get to their offices tomorrow and sign the paperwork," I said.

"Well, I think that at this point, you've done everything that you can and should have. Everything's documented, and you've filled out a police report, which is exactly what your attorney is going to want to start with. What St. Louis County is going to do or is willing to do, I simply don't know," he said. "Do you have anything else that you want to add to the police report? Was there any physical violence involved?"

"No, there was no physical violence involved. I've never even touched a woman in that manner before and never would, and my mother can testify to that fact. I only have one other thing to add. She had a fucking padlock screwed in her bedroom door. Whoever came over to steal the furniture busted the door off its hinges. They must have been so stupid as to lose the key. There's substantial damage," I said.

"OK, well, here's the number of your police report, and it will be formalized and in our system come Monday or Tuesday afternoon. That's when your attorney will be able to get a copy of it. If you need anything further, just give us a call, especially if she or anyone on that side of the family shows up at your door over the weekend," he said.

"So basically there's nothing that you're going to do, right?" I asked.

"Well, she's really not committed any crimes to speak of," the deputy replied.

I couldn't leave well enough alone. "So you're telling me that even kidnapping my kids is not a crime?"

"Are they legally her kids also?" the deputy asked.

"Yes," I replied.

"Then she has just as much right to see them as you do," he replied.

"Then what I'm hearing is that I have just as much right to go over to her in-laws and get my kids back, right?"I asked.

"Technically, yes, but if you cause any disturbance whatsoever, your in-laws are going to call St. Louis

County Police and try to have you arrested. That's a road that I wouldn't go down if I were you. I would wait until you get the proper legal advice from your attorney," the deputy responded.

"OK, thanks for your help, and I'll call with any further problems," I said. I couldn't get it out of my head that kidnapping was legal for the wife but illegal for the husband!

As it turned out, my wife had already moved into an apartment in St. Louis County not that far from her parents' house. I found out this information from my nanny who still had half a heart left. She called me later that evening to tell me everything that had transpired during the day. Half of my furniture was already neatly moved into her new apartment, and apparently she had quite a bit of help given the timing. My kids were already going to private school, and she found a new carpool for them and just went on with life like nothing had ever happened. My two youngest kids were way too young to understand what had happened or where their dad had gone. To them, I was a deadbeat father; I had walked out on them and left them living in a cheap-ass apartment, sleeping in a cramped room together. I pray that through this book and the many discussions that I have had with them they will never forget the truth.

There are casualties in any war, and unfortunately for them, my children found themselves casualties of the war named divorce, the big *D* that further unraveled over the course of not just months but years. In total, my divorce has lasted seven years and counting. Family, friends, colleagues, and doctors all ask the same question: How is that even possible? I have a single-word answer: greed. What I went through, what my children went through, and everything we lost, I would not wish upon my worst enemy for any reason. I am not free of guilt, and I have never claimed to be. However, I did not set the tone for this divorce from the beginning.

I don't know what happened to the blocks of time that I seem to have lost so effortlessly, time that had been erased from my mind like a hard drive from a computer. I've questioned my friends, I've questioned my family, I've even questioned my own children. I'm stuck now in an endless loop like Earth circling the sun. I have finally awakened from this maddening nightmare and found that I still call my own kids children even though their ages dictate otherwise.

On May 7, 2009, my divorce was finalized only to the extent that both of us signed the divorce papers. Little did I know that the date only marked the beginning of the end of a portion of my life. This date also marked the end of my ambulatory period. The stress alone from going through a divorce and losing everything that I had spent a lifetime building caused a massive exacerbation that not even massive doses of steroids could pull me out of. A few months after my divorce was finalized, I had to throw out my walker in lieu of my new transportation method—a manual wheelchair.

Utilizing a manual wheelchair meant that I had lost the use of my legs altogether. This in turn meant that I had to have my car modified with a manual hand brake and gas device as I could no longer use the foot pedals. Looking back on it now, I seemed to take it all in stride, Probably because no matter how angry I was or how much revenge I sought, there simply was nothing I could do but sit back and watch my body further deteriorate.

It was a period of great consternation for myself and one in which I found myself in an extremely depressive state of mind. Luckily for me, I understood what this meant and the risk I ran for suicide, therefore I wasted no time in going back to my psychiatrist for an adjustment in medications.

My ex-wife held the advantage over me in this disheartening melodrama. Every day of my life, I prayed for the opportunity to not relive my life but to simply have dreams where I recalled happier days and could watch my children grow and hear their voices and laughter.

I wish I understood then what I know now, for the lives of my children would have turned out so different-ly—of this I am confident. While my marriage turned out to be a statistical fluke, there was so much more to it than I could ever put to words. I have gaps in my memory that span nearly half a decade, memories of my children that are gone like flames in a fire. I see the questions on their precious faces, the questions they are afraid to ask but that I am well aware of. Questions that their mother has rammed down their throats and stuffed into their ears to the point where they believed I was the devil incarnate. How do you ever begin to get children to believe right from wrong? How do you ever get children to believe that one of their parents could actually be wrong in the first place? Where were you, Father? Where were you during my childhood? Why weren't you at my games, Dad? Why weren't you at my graduation, Father? I cried, I prayed, I asked Christ for their understanding and forgiveness. I prayed to Him for this strength I so desperately needed to face this world alone and be with my children for the rest of their days. I prayed to Christ that He would not allow me to slip and fall again. I have, for the first time, gained the traction that I so desperately need to keep pace with my children and their lives. Now is not the time to wallow in self-pity. Now is the time to rejoice in what has been given me even though the losses still outweigh the gains, I will not complain.

I live alone now, the progression of my disease over the past several years has required that I have nearly full-time assistance to do even the most basic things in life; things I once did without thought. Our house is gone now. What once stood as a symbol of the strength of our family has come crumbling down. I had to dump it in a recession and barely made back the buckets of money I made when I sold my house in Chicago. It's not about the money, I could really care less as it's more about the personal life I lost; the money I can make back.

CARPET BOMBING

*It doesn't take a hero to order men
into battle. It takes a hero to be one of
those men who goes into battle.*

— Norman Schwarzkopf

January 10, 2015.

Years of my life had vanished in a hurricane that was my disaster of a divorce, and now, another year of my life was about to disappear in the thickest of London fogs, and I was ill-prepared. Never in the twenty-five years of battling this miserable disease, had I ever been punched in the gut as hard as I was about to be. I found myself in the trenches of war with mortar rounds exploding yards from where I lay. The thickest sheets of armor would have failed to protect me. Again I questioned whether I simply missed the warning signs or just chose to ignore them altogether. I prayed for death this time, to whom I know not but a shadow of something much worse came to visit, and I alone bore witness to its hideousness. Life could not be so kind as to give you your five minute break. Whether others believe or not, I don't care—I now know the face of true evil.

I awoke Saturday morning in the ICU at Mercy Hospital at around eight o'clock. I found myself lying flat on my back, staring straight up at a massive surgical lamp that had been pulled down from the ceiling to within a few feet of my chest. The lamp was luminous, and I instinctively shut my eyes intensely to avoid it. I instantly began to panic and tried in vain to throw the blankets off of me, but my arms would not respond. I had somehow transformed from being a paraplegic to a quadriplegic overnight—or was it overnight? How long had I been lying here? I thought of my hero, Christopher Reeve; I had become him.

A tear ran down my cheek and settled on the lobe of my ear. Where were the nurses, the doctors? Why was no one helping me? I started to yell, but before I could, a pulse-rate alarm went off on one of the many monitors hooked up to me. I knew that my rate had to be over a hundred beats per minute. No sooner did the alarm go off than a group of nurses and a doctor entered the room or space that I occupied.

The doctor reached up over my head and shut the alarm off. "Michael, can you hear me talking?" the doctor asked while giving me a cursory eye exam with his penlight.

I responded yes with a raspy voice.

"Michael, you're a pretty sick man right now, but we have everything under control, OK?" the doctor said.

"OK. When will you tell me what exactly happened to me? I can't even move my arms or my hands anymore. Was I running a fever? If so, I'm sure I'm experiencing an exacerbation. Have you contacted my neurologist? I need to be on Solu-Medrol as soon as possible," I said. I knew the importance of getting the Solu-Medrol into my system as I would not be able to function properly without it. Solu-Medrol is basically a high dose IV steroid which when given to MS patients during an exacerbation, basically stops the nerve swelling within the central nervous system.

I noted that my parents were not in the room with me. Because of the time, I assumed that they were probably at home asleep.

"Do you remember what happened yesterday, Michael?" the doctor asked.

My mind was racing a mile a minute, but I knew this routine. "No, I don't remember anything at all," I responded.

"Do you know your last name, Michael?" The doctor asked.

"Yes, Seliner," I replied. "The current president is Obama; I'm at Mercy Hospital; I know it's nighttime, but I don't know either the day or the date," I said.

"OK, well, you were brought in about ten o'clock Saturday evening with a fever of one hundred and five. You were unconscious, and unresponsive; we could not wake you up," he said. "It's good to see that you've recovered so quickly."

"Do you know what I have? Was it a UTI?" I asked.

"Yeah, it was a UTI, and a pretty nasty one at that. We're still letting the cultures run their course, but from what we've seen so far, we've had to put you on two of our big-gun antibiotics," he said. "The paramedics who brought you in this morning reported that they had found you lying in a pool of blood with a very high fever. They further indicated that they could not wake you up, and that's how you ended up here."

A nurse came over to my bedside and told me that she had called my parents, who said that they would be on their way back up shortly. I felt like I had been run over by a Mack truck. Every bone in my body ached. If I had a way to get a hold of my morphine, I would've swallowed half the bottle, but that wasn't the case, was it? Nope, from here on out all my drugs would be strictly regimented by the ER doctors, which completely sucked. I was the patient; didn't

I know what was best for me? Another freaking stay in the hospital, and this one was turning out to be a doozy. How long—one week, two weeks, maybe more?

I only recognized the hospital that I was in by the uniforms the nurses were wearing; my glasses had been removed, but I had been there plenty of times before. I was what they called a regular here at Mercy.

It was difficult to try to draw in a deep breath of air; my sinuses were impacted. I must have had an oxygen meter on my finger, and it must have been reading below 92 percent, as one of the nurses kept asking me to take a few deep breaths.

"Are you having trouble breathing, Michael?" the doctor asked.

"Yes. I can't breathe through my nose; it's completely impacted. I feel like there's a person sitting on my chest," I said.

"Have you ever had any heart problems before, Michael?" he asked.

"No, none whatsoever," I responded.

"Let's get respiratory up here to take a look at him, and make sure they bring a breathing treatment also," the doctor said to one of the nurses. "Janet, since he's having problems breathing through his nose, let's get a full mask on him, and I want that with four liters, OK?"

Janet, one of the nurses, took the cannula out of my nose and put a full mask over my nose and mouth, and then cranked up the oxygen to four liters. It felt nothing short of liberating to be able to breathe again.

"How's that feel, Michael? Better or worse?"

"Much better," I mumbled through the mask.

"OK, good. Respiratory is going to be here within a few minutes, and they're going to give you a breathing treatment, which is just a dose of albuterol. Have you had albuterol before?" the doctor asked.

"Yeah, no problems with it," I responded.

The doctor walked up to the side of my bed and said, "Just lay here and try to relax, Michael. You're going to be OK. Like I said, respiratory will be here within a few minutes, and in the meantime, we're going to try to find you a room as I feel that you need to be admitted, OK? Any questions?" he asked.

Admittedly, I had a ton of questions, but I knew that the last thing that he wanted to do was sit there and answer them. I could just as easily get my answers from one of the many nurses within the room. I would wait. "No, I'm fine for now, thanks," I responded.

Another alarm on one of the monitors began beeping. This was a serious one, and one that the doctor was not so quick to simply dismiss. My oxygen saturation had fallen below 85 percent and was decreasing by the minute. He asked me if I was having trouble breathing. I told him I was and that I needed to sit up as quickly as possible. He went over to the phone and must've called respiratory stat.

Within seconds, the room was filled with at least five nurses and doctors from the respiratory department. They quickly checked the level of oxygen that I was on and confirmed it with the doctor. They too asked me if I was having problems breathing, to which I responded that my chest felt tight. One of the doctors suggested that I must have a plugged air duct in my left lung as my breathing sounds were very decreased. He immediately ordered the oxygen level to be increased to seven liters with albuterol and that they start quad coughing stat.

"Do you know what quad coughing is, Mike?" the doctor asked.

"No," I mumbled the best I could through the high volume of air that was blowing into my lungs.

"We believe you have a mucus-plugged airway, and we need to clear it out immediately," the doctor said. "Quad coughing sounds a lot more complex than it actually is. To put it simply, one of the nurses is going to help you to cough by pushing on your left lung at the same time you try to cough," he said. "Are you ready to give this a try?"

This time, I simply nodded my head as I was growing very tired.

"Okay, on the count of three, try to cough as hard as you can at the same time. The nurse will assist you," the doctor said.

On the count of three, I felt a massive push by the nurse on my lung that completely overcame my weak attempt to cough. I felt an immediate rush of air into my left lung, and within seconds, my oxygen meter stopped beeping. I could once again smell and taste the albuterol as it rushed through my respiratory system.

Why was I here? What happened to me? At first I thought I must have had a stroke or another pulmonary embolism (PE), but I was already on a chronic dose of a blood thinner, warfarin, and had been for some time. Maybe my INR number had dipped below therapeutic or shot above for that matter, causing me to bleed internally. Certainly they would've picked up on that, I thought. With oxygen, the fog in my head lifted slightly, but my voice was still raspy. *Jesus, is this what has become of me? Did I fall victim to a massive stroke?*

My clothes had been removed and replaced with a hospital gown—another freaking gown to add to my collection. I think I'll open up a thrift store for medical supplies. I could not move my arms or even bend my fingers. My body lay buried under three layers of blankets, and I didn't want a single one of them. I was burning up. How did I become a quadriplegic? It had to be due to an exacerbation from the high fever. I tried to replay the events that took place prior to me awakening at the hospital, but there was nothing but darkness, emptiness; my memory had been wiped clean. My memory had failed me. Something was seriously wrong, and I had the feeling that they were waiting for my parents to show up before telling me the bad news.

"I already called your mother, and your parents are on their way back up now," said one of the nurses. Someone else had already told me that bit of information, right?

"Can you please remove the blankets?" I asked. My eyelids were heavy with sleep, and I blinked slowly. My voice was also slow and raspy. These facts do not go unnoticed by the doctor; he asked one of the nurses to chart it.

"Do you want them partway down or all the way off?" she asked.

"All the way off, please. I'm burning up," I responded. "Can I ask? Did I have a stroke or a PE?"

"No, the CAT scans did not reveal anything except for some fluid in your lungs, which is probably the onset of pneumonia," she responded. She further indicated that the pneumonia was most likely one of the reasons why I was having problems breathing. I asked the nurse if she could turn down the air inside my room; my forehead was sweating. She quickly took my temperature again, and it was at 101.5 degrees Fahrenheit. "Yeah, you still have a low-grade fever. I'm going to ask if I can get you some Tylenol, OK?" she asked.

"OK," I responded, "and please turn off the overhead lamp," I said.

"I'll be back in a few minutes; just hit the call button if there's anything that you need," she said.

"I can't use my arms or hands and, therefore, can't push the call button. Is there something else that you could hook up for me?" I asked.

"Yeah, we have an air-blow system that we could hook up rather quickly for you. All you'll have to do is blow real lightly into the pipe that we can bend up right by your mouth, and that will signal a nurse to come. Let me get everything together that I need and get one of the other nurses to help me first, OK?" she asked.

I lay on the bed with a hospital gown on and a single pillow under my head, which was cocked to the left, but I could not move my head to center it back on the pillow. I broke down and started crying like a child. Memories of riding my motorcycle in Denver crept into my head, and a smile slowly came across my face. Freedom—freedom from everything and everyone. There simply was nothing like it, and now I had been robbed of it. I didn't care who was in the room at that point; I was severely broken and worried that no one could fix me. I prayed intensely for my family to walk in the door. My mother would know immediately what to do—she always knew what to do.

I just wanted to be back home more than anything as I knew this hospital stay was going to be longer than normal, and I was simply too worn down to put up a fight. I opened my mouth, but the words didn't come out; I choked. One of the nurses came over and handed me a box of tissues. The other nurse told her that I couldn't move my arms and that she would have to wipe my eyes. I stared intently into her eyes as she did it. She was embarrassed and tried to look away. I was a forty-seven-year-old broken-down man who could not turn the faucet off—a mind with no body. She kindly wiped my eyes for me and then repositioned my head on the center of the pillow. Death would've been a welcome friend.

Another nurse entered the room with a bag of Solu-Medrol to hang. My old friend, I thought. I then realized that true help in the way of pharmaceuticals was on the way and that it would only be a matter of hours now before I felt its effect. I lay on the table and closed my eyes just waiting for that heavy taste of copper to fill my mouth. I knew that once I tasted the copper pennies, it would only be a matter of a couple of hours before I would be able to move my arms again. Who cares if autoimmune diseases are only treated with steroids? They work.

At around noon, my parents entered my room, set down their belongings, and came over to my side. "Are you thirsty, honey? Do you want anything to drink?" my mother asked.

An immediate sense of relief rushed over my body and mind. I knew now that no matter what, I would be okay; my parents would fix me better than any doctor could.

"Yeah, dying of thirst. I would love an ice-cold water. Would you mind going down to the cafeteria to get me one?" I responded. "How did I end up getting admitted so late on Friday?" I asked my father.

"Well, you told your mother that you weren't feeling too well earlier in the evening on Friday, and when she checked your temperature, she found out that you had a low-grade fever," he responded.

"So did she end up staying awake with me all night or what?" I asked.

"No, she came up to bed at her normal time, around ten o'clock, but she kept going downstairs to check on you until your temperature had gone up to one hundred and two. Apparently she tried to wake you up to give you some more Tylenol, and when she pulled your blanket back, she noticed that you were sitting in a pool of blood," he said.

"Pool of blood?" I asked, shocked.

"Yeah, that's what I understand, and from what we learned last night when you were admitted, you had a UTI and they thought it was bad enough to cause you to urinate blood. You really need to talk to your mother, Mike, if you want to know more details. I'm sorry, but you know me and hospitals—we just don't get along," he said.

Just then my mother came in with a large ice water. and one of the nurses walked in behind her. My mom asked if it was OK if I had some ice water to drink, and the nurse had no problem with it. My mother gave me the water and then proceeded to look over the bags of medicine that were hanging up on the pole above my bed. "What's Solu-Medrol?" she asked.

"It's a pretty powerful steroid that helps to stop or slow down the swelling of many different things, not the least of which are nerves in my body," I said. "So can you fill me in on what happened last night? What did you think or do when you saw that I was sitting in a pool of blood in my recliner?"

"Well, I was absolutely shocked and scared to death so I immediately called nine-one-one and told them what was going on. I don't think I've ever seen them come out to the house so quickly. They had their lights on, and there must have been, geez, six of them inside the house," she responded.

"So they probably didn't even do anything once they got there, did they?" I asked.

"Well, I remember them taking your vitals while they were trying to wake you up, which I couldn't do. One of the paramedics told me that they had even tried to perform…I think it's called a sternum rub…and that didn't even work. After that, they immediately loaded you up onto the stretcher, and they were gone. I mean, they didn't even sit outside like they normally do for a few minutes before leaving," she said.

"Certainly you didn't follow them all the way up here last night, did you?" I asked.

"Of course I did; what else was I supposed to do?" she said.

"So what did they tell you was going on with me after you got here?" I asked.

"For the longest time they really didn't say anything, but I think that was just because they honestly didn't know. They did tell me that they were drawing blood for labs and doing cultures. How long have you been awake now?" she asked.

"I don't recall, maybe since about eight o'clock or so. I remember the nurse telling me that they had already been in contact with you and that was shortly after I woke up, I think," I said. "I have to be honest, I really don't feel all that bad right now, but my buttocks are extremely painful, and I'm more worried about those sores than anything. I wish the wound nurses would get in here soon and take a look at them."

"I told them that you had two pressure ulcers on your backside when I got here last night, and they told me that they would take a look at them; I guess they haven't followed up with that yet," she said.

"Nope, still waiting," I said.

Around noon, a nurse came in and told us that I was being admitted and would be going to the hospital's step-down unit, which is apparently where patients go once they get released from the ICU. My parents were both relieved that I was being released from the ICU, and I have to admit that I felt I was one step closer to going back home, hopefully within a day or two. My parents stayed with me until the transport team came and picked me up, and then followed us to the step-down unit where they had a room ready for me.

Once I got hooked back up to everything and transported over to my new low air-loss mattress, they let me be for a while, probably to let me have a chance to talk with my parents a bit more.

"So I guess there's been no talk as of yet about when you may be released from the hospital?" my mom asked.

"No, they haven't said anything to that effect, but knowing how long cultures take to grow, I would assume that I'm going to be here for at least three to four days," I replied.

My mother was in the middle of making small talk about some of the things that she had to do like getting her hair done when the wound nurses walked in and asked if they could have a moment. I asked them if I could say good-bye to my parents first, which they were fine with. I hugged and kissed my mother and gave my dad a firm handshake as usual. This was a routine that all of us were more than accustomed to.

"I'll call you later on this evening, honey, but if you need anything in the meantime, give me a shout, OK? I'll be back up tomorrow, but I won't have the opportunity to get here until after noon. Is that OK?" she asked.

"Mom, that's fine. Don't rush to get up here. Feel free to come up later in the day. I'll be fine, and if I hear any further news I'll give you a call, OK?" I asked.

"OK, honey. We love you very much, and hopefully you get to leave here soon," my mother said.

"OK, see ya, sport. You hang in there, OK?" my dad said.

My mother grabbed another kiss from me before both of them walked out the door and headed down the hall. I was sad to see them go.

The wound nurses had been waiting outside in the hallway. "Hi, my name is Nancy, and this is Rebecca, and we are wound nurses from the wound clinic here at Mercy. We understand that you have two pressure ulcers on your buttocks that we need to take a look at. Is that correct?" Nancy asked. "By the way, I'm sorry—do you go by Mike or Michael?"

A grin came across my face. "Mike's fine," I replied.

"Can you tell us how long you've had these sores?" Rebecca asked.

I went on to tell them that I'd had the sores for approximately four weeks and that my mother and a home-health nurse had been cleaning them and bandaging them twice a day. I was asked what I did for a living, how much time I spent sitting in my wheelchair per day, and if I had a low air-loss mattress like the one I was on at home.

"I'm a mechanical engineer by trade, and I would say that I probably spend about ten hours per day at work just sitting in my wheelchair. Then I go home and sit down in my leather recliner where I also sleep. I don't have a low air-loss mattress at home, and my regular bed mattress is too hard for me to sleep on," I said.

"And are you a paraplegic?" Nancy asked.

"Yes, I am, but I do have about eighty percent feeling below the waist," I responded.

"So you're pretty much on your bottom for most of the day, correct?" she asked.

"Yep, unfortunately that's right. Currently I have no way of transferring out of my wheelchair except for a wooden transfer board that I try to avoid as much as possible because of all the pain it causes with my sores," I said.

"We're going to need to take measurements of the sores in order to document them and to best know how to treat them, OK?" Rebecca said.

"OK, that's fine," I responded.

"Mike, it looks like the one pressure ulcer that you have on your right side is pretty deep right now, and the one on your left side is only about half the size as the one on your right," Nancy said.

"Can I ask you what exactly you'll do differently than how I am taking care of them at home?" I asked.

"Sure. Right now the main thing that we're going to do differently is clean the sores thoroughly, which involves getting rid of all the dead skin and tissue inside the ulcer itself. A lot of times, people just clean the wounds and bandage them, and that's OK as long as you're not continuing to apply pressure to the ulcers, which, in your case, seems like an impossibility," Rebecca said.

"Does that make sense, Mike?" Nancy asked. "A lot of times, what happens is that these sores begin tunneling into new tissue, and that's how they continue to grow in size. Sometimes sores like these will get to the point that a plastic surgeon will have to do what is called a flap surgery, which is where they basically close up the wounds because our methods of treatment are too superficial and no longer help to heal the wound."

"In addition, Mike, we're going to have to add you to what's called the turn team, which is a team of nurses' assistants that will come in every two hours and rotate you from one side of your body to the other," Rebecca said. "This will help us to ensure that we have you completely off of your bottom and that we are allowing the sores to heal properly. If we can't get them to heal properly, as Nancy was saying, that's when a plastic surgeon will get called in to perform the flap surgery, which is something that we can hopefully avoid."

As it turned out, the nurses had found that there was tunneling in both pressure ulcers and that they would have to clean them on a daily basis until all of the dead skin and tissue was gone; I had no idea what was in store for me. They had no idea how deep the tunneling would go. We would both find out at the same time.

The following morning, breakfast had just shown up when I was visited by therapists from occupational therapy, physical therapy, and speech therapy. I was familiar with the routine of therapy, but never before had I been visited by therapists so soon after I had been admitted. The reason they gave for being there so soon was related to the fact that I had spiked such a high fever in addition to the paralysis I experienced. The speech therapist, whom I had never worked with before, started by asking me several questions to check my cognitive functions.

"Mike, my name's Karen, and I'm a speech therapist. Do you know where you are right now?" she asked.

"Mercy Hospital," I responded.

"Good, and can you tell me why you're here?" she asked.

"Well, from what I've been told, I spiked a very high fever and became unconscious," I said.

"Good, that's right. Now can you tell me what day it is?" she asked.

"No, I honestly have no idea," I said.

"OK, that's all right. Can you tell me what year it is?" she asked.

"Two thousand fifteen?" I responded hesitantly.

"You didn't sound too sure of yourself on that answer. Do you know if it is two thousand fifteen for sure?" she asked.

"Yes, it's two thousand fifteen. I'm sure," I responded.

"OK, thanks," she said. "I have about ten mathematical flashcards, each of which I'm going to show you for a period of approximately ten seconds, and I want you to give me the answer to them, OK?" she asked.

"Are these equations ones that I'm supposed to do in my head?" I asked.

"That's right; these are just like the old flashcards that you used to do in grade school. They involve just the basics, which are addition and subtraction and multiplication and division, OK?" she replied.

I still recall laughing about that because engineering was my expertise, and mathematical problems are normally a breeze for me. Since Karen from speech therapy had shown up prior to the other two ladies from occupational and physical therapy, she stayed to finish her evaluation while the other two ladies indicated that they would be back within an hour.

As Karen was getting her flashcards together, I stared out the window of my fifth-floor room to a roof stack that was apparently venting hot air. The cloud it formed continued to grow and dissipate as I wondered how cold it was outside.

Karen interrupted me when she started asking me for answers to the mathematical equations. I instantly began having trouble thinking or remembering how to do the problems. I gave Karen a half-assed attempt at a laugh, telling her that I didn't know what exactly was wrong with me, that normally math problems like those should have been no problem. Five times five equals…how could I not know the answer to this? I was completely embarrassed that I couldn't even do this simple problem.

Karen was actually very understanding about my issue and went on to explain that was why she was there—it can sometimes be difficult for people who have spiked a very high fever and have gone unconscious to perform what we would normally consider simple or mundane tasks. She went on for the following hour tormenting me, performing several different tests, all of which were aimed at testing my current cognitive state. Since it was quite alarming to me how poorly I had done, I asked her how much therapy I would be receiving, especially if I did not show improvement by the time I was over my pneumonia. She indicated that the hospital had special off-site therapy facilities where I could go as either an in- or outpatient and receive continued therapy until my cognitive skills were back to normal.

The occupational and physical therapists came back within a half hour after Karen left, and they mainly worked with me in trying to build my strength back up from the upper-body paralysis that I had experienced. Even though I had been on high-dose IV steroids, I still had not regained full function of my upper body. This minor detail bothered me as I had never experienced it before—my strength had always come back immediately. The plan was for me to work with them, just like Karen, for the duration of my stay at the hospital.

My attending doctor, Dr. Bhatia, came in and visited with me at around two o'clock. Dr. Bhatia started things off by talking to me about my condition, my current ailments, and how they were going to treat each one.

"Mr. Seliner, you were admitted to the hospital late Friday night, and you were unconscious at the time. We're not one hundred percent sure at this time why you were unconscious, but we believe that it was due to your high fever. In any event, we'll be running some additional tests to verify or rule out anything serious that we need to be treating besides what we're already aware of," Dr. Bhatia said.

"Doctor, I have a quick question," I said. "I miserably failed a bunch of simple mathematical equations, and I'm talking about addition and subtraction here, with the speech therapist this morning. How concerned should I be about the long-term effects of the high fever that I spiked, and do you think that I will be going to in- or outpatient therapy after I leave this hospital?"

"Well, to answer the first part of your question, we rarely see long-term effects of patients spiking a fever except in cases where we were unable to get the fever under control within a few hours or in the very young or very old. In your case, I really don't foresee any long-term issues, although I'm sure that you probably will struggle for a week or so. I would not get yourself too worked up over your current situation. I know it can be scary, but you just need to get over that and concentrate on the work at hand. Keeping your focus will help you bring back those functions that you have temporarily lost.

"To answer the second part of your question, we first need to make the determination that you will even require further therapy upon discharge from the hospital. It may be that you will require no further help, but if you do, you will have a choice of going to either inpatient or outpatient therapy. I'm sure that your insurance company will be heavily involved in that decision. Does that answer your questions?" he asked.

"Yes, it does, thank you," I said.

Dr. Bhatia further explained that they were somewhat concerned about my pressure ulcers, and that treatment of those might be a little trickier than treatment of pneumonia. Pneumonia usually responds well to medications, but there were no medications to close up pressure ulcers. He said that they would have to wait and see how things looked over the next four days or so. "Did the wound nurses get a chance to evaluate you yet?" he asked.

"Yeah, they came by and measured the sores and photographed them. They basically told me the same thing that you just did. From what they found, it sounds like the sores may be in worse condition than I thought," I said.

"OK, then you know what we'll be looking for over the next few days as we track their progress. Do you have any other questions for me?" he asked.

"No, but thank you very much. I appreciate your time," I replied.

Five days after initially being admitted to the hospital, I was released with the suggestion from my doctors that I attend further inpatient therapy programs because I was still experiencing some strength and speech issues and the pressure ulcers were not fully healed. It was worked out between my family and my insurance company that I would be moved directly to Mercy Hospital's inpatient therapy facility for a maximum period of four weeks.

During my stay there, I was fortunate enough to regain all my faculties, but my pressure ulcers continued to get worse. Prior to my discharge, my attending physician visited to take a look at them and make a decision on what to do.

"Mr. Seliner, I hate to be the one to deliver bad news under any circumstances, but I feel that we really need to operate on these wounds upon discharge," Dr. Bhatia said. "I've consulted with the wound clinic, and while they feel that they finally have the growth of the pressure ulcers under control, they have no plan going forward on how to close them up without plastic surgery. Right now, your largest sore is on your right side, and it measures three inches in diameter by two and a half inches deep. Under any circumstance, this would be considered a massive open injury that needs to be closed up. The good news is that the skin on the sores is completely healed now, which means that the plastic surgeon will have more to work with when closing up the sores. Does that make sense?"

"OK, so can you explain to me exactly what he'll do?" I asked.

"Well, that's going to be completely up to the particular plastic surgeon who performs the surgery, but in essence, they're simply going to close the wounds up using a technique called a flap surgery. You obviously have your choice of both doctors and hospitals, and that's a decision that you're going to need to make here over the next couple of days before we release you. Ideally, what we'd like to see happen is for you to be transferred directly from this facility to whichever hospital you decide to have the surgery at," he said.

"Well, then, I'll talk with my family and make a decision and let you know what our plans are before I get discharged from here, OK?" I said.

"OK, that sounds fine by me. Just make sure that you're also in touch with the wound nurses," he said.

After speaking with my PCP, I decided to have my flap surgery performed by Dr. Kloch at Saint Anthony's Hospital in St. Louis. Dr. Kloch was a friend of my PCP, and he trusted him, which made my decision quite easy. After advising the staff at Mercy Hospital, I was immediately transferred via ambulance to Saint Anthony's Hospital. Upon being admitted, Dr. Kloch stopped by my room to introduce himself and go over the surgery.

"Mr. Seliner, my name's Dr. Kloch. I believe you know me through your PCP, Dr. Mason, is that correct?" he asked with a smile. Dr. Kloch seemed like an ordinary guy, and had he not been wearing his doctor's coat, I never would've known that he was an accomplished plastic surgeon. I immediately understood why he and Dr. Mason were good friends. I was put at ease and felt like I was talking to a good friend also.

"Yeah, Dr. Mason has been my doctor for more years than I can count. He recommended you for this surgery, and I trust him completely. Plus, he said you would take good care of me," I said laughingly.

"Well, you've got nothing to worry about. I will take good care you, on that you have my promise. The reason I stopped by was because I wanted to get a good look at your pressure ulcers. Is that OK?" he asked.

"Yeah, no problem," I said.

Dr. Kloch proceeded to take measurements and photographs of what was left of my pressure ulcers. He told me that a full flap surgery would not be required and that he would most likely be stitching them closed from the inside out. He also told me that he had booked surgery for the following morning, which kind of surprised me at first, but after thinking about it, I was glad.

"I see that you're still on a bunch of IV medications. Is that still related to the pneumonia that you were diagnosed with?" he asked.

"That's correct. I started to turn the corner in regard to the pneumonia, but then it came back within a week after they took me off the meds, so they decided to put me back on for another couple weeks just in case. They didn't want it coming back, and I certainly agreed with them," I replied.

"OK, the surgery itself is going to take me about two and a half hours as long as I don't encounter any issues, which I don't plan on at this point. The worst part is not going to be the surgery as much as the post-op care. Did anyone talk to you about how long total recovery would take and what it involves?" he asked.

"No, I didn't speak to anyone about it," I said.

"Well, total recovery is going to take anywhere from eight to ten weeks. The worst part is that you're going to have to spend those eight to ten weeks off your back and on your sides. You're familiar with the turn teams, are you not?" he asked.

I never heard him ask me any questions. I was still in shock about the eight- to ten-week recovery period. *You've got to be fucking kidding me,* I thought. There was simply no way that I could go through with this. What was I supposed to do, tell him that I was canceling the surgery and go home?

"Mr. Seliner, you still with me?" he asked.

"Yeah, I'm here. Sorry. I was just thinking about the total length of the recovery period. I just honestly don't know how I'm going to be able to pull this one off," I said apologetically.

"I completely understand, and the only thing I can tell you is to surround yourself with friends and family and purchase a bunch of electronic toys beforehand. Trust me; you'll be surprised at how tough your mind can actually be. You'll make it through this; you need to make it through this," he said. "It was good to meet you, Mr. Seliner, and I'll be seeing you again tomorrow morning at seven o'clock sharp for the surgery, OK?"

"OK, Dr. Kloch. Thanks again, and I'll see you in the morning," I said.

Two days after a successful surgery to close up my pressure ulcers, I developed C-diff from overuse of the antibiotics that were being given to me to fight my previous infections; ironically. This was a serious and unforeseen complication that jeopardized the success of my surgery. Dr. Kloch came in the day after I was diagnosed diff and told me that they would not be able to stop the infection until after my wounds from the surgery healed. His main concern was that my post-op wounds would become infected, which was a situation that he indicated he did not want to see happen but that could happen quite easily.

"Dr. Kloch, what are my options outside of the medications that they are already giving me to fight the C-diff?" I asked.

"I hate to be the one to tell you this, Mike, but there's really no way around this. You need a colostomy. I can only imagine what your initial thoughts are and what's going through your mind right now, but we can do what's called a partial colostomy that can be reversed once everything is healed. If you decide that you don't want to keep the colostomy, we can always simply undo it. So, all in all, it may seem like a horrible thing to have to go through, but you need to keep in mind that it can be reversed. We're not talking about anything permanent here, OK?" he said.

I still recall my emotional state right after he told me that I would need a colostomy—total disbelief and anger. For the remainder of that afternoon and well into the evening, I consulted with family and friends who were all supportive and quick to point out that the colostomy was reversible. I spoke with Dr. Kloch the following morning and gave him permission to perform the surgery.

He introduced me to one of his colleagues who was a gastrointestinal surgeon and would be performing the actual surgery. He informed me that because of my infection, they needed to move quickly and that he would schedule surgery for later that afternoon.

I woke up the next morning, looked at what the surgeon had done, and simply broke down in tears. I would go so far as to say that I was near hysterical and simply wanted to go home, which I could not. Several of my regular nurses at the hospital came in and talked to me to try to get me to calm down, and I was very appreciative of their actions as I'm not sure if I could have pulled out of my emotional slip without their help.

During my recovery at the hospital, I was mainly immobile for a period of no less than eight weeks. I was told that because of the location of the sores, I would not receive physical or occupational therapy during that time frame as they did not want the wounds to open up again. Basically, I couldn't sit or lie on my back because I would be putting pressure on my buttocks. I felt betrayed, I felt like I had been lied to.

So Kindred Hospital, which was on the campus of Saint Anthony's, was my home for eight weeks, during which I would not be able to leave the room, have any physical exercise whatsoever, and could have no person-to-person interaction, as C-diff is a highly contagious disease. Prison—hell, solitary confinement would have been better.

After four continuous months in the hospital, my insurance ran out, and I had to be relocated from Kindred Hospital to Green Park Nursing Home, where I was to receive my final four weeks of rehabilitation and physical and occupational therapy. The problem, however, as it was presented to me was that my wounds still needed a couple more weeks of healing before I could begin any type of therapy. I ended up waiting for a total of eighteen weeks before they started physical and occupational therapy. I was also told that I would only receive two weeks of therapy due to the fact that my insurance was yet again running out and that after this stay, the only other option I had was to head home where I would have to pay out-of-pocket for the remainder of my required therapies.

After a total of twenty continuous weeks in the hospital, I had lost over forty-five pounds of fat and muscle and was atrophied from being immobilized for so long. I felt like a piece of garbage that no one knew what to do with. I felt that death would've been better, and I wished for it to come knocking on my door.

Both doctors and nurses alike say that for every week that you spend in the hospital recovering from a surgery, you should expect to spend three additional weeks in occupational and physical therapy. For me, this equation meant that I should have spent sixty weeks in therapy and this was for occupational and physical therapy only. In all honesty, I should have spent additional time in speech therapy, at least enough time to help properly clear my head as my thoughts were still fuzzy. Instead I spent only two weeks due to insurance, due to a flow chart that sat on some insurance adjuster's desk.

I knew that if I had any hope of getting back to where I was before my incident, I would have to put in the personal time and effort without the use of hospital staff.

At my own expense, I began working with a Certified Nursing Assistant (CNA) for a period of eight hours per day for 25 weeks while back at home. It was once again that I learned all of the basic life functions that I had so quickly forgotten or lost during my stay in the hospital.

CLOSING TIME

January 25, 2016.

"So, Mike, I received your message. Last session together, huh?" Bob asked. "You sure you're ready?"

"Come on, Bob, you know you're just trying to drum up more business," I said.

"No, you know that's not it. I just want to make sure that you're going to be OK and I want you to know that you're always welcome to get in touch with me and j chat if you'd like; of course e-mails are always free," Bob said.

"Do you know what General Patton said about courage, Bob?" I asked.

"No, what's that?" Bob replied.

"He said, 'Courage is fear holding on a minute longer.' I have to say that I've never heard so much truth spoken in a single sentence," I said. "You know, I've been giving it some thought, and I'd like for you to start calling me Michael, if you don't mind." I imagined a big grin coming across Bob's face, followed by laughter.

"To be honest with you, I always liked the name Michael better for some reason. I thank you for that, and for our last session together, I will call you, Michael," Bob replied. "I saw that you booked two sessions back-to-back. Is there a problem I need to be made aware of, or do you just have a lot on your mind?"

I responded by telling him that there really was no problem, but I felt that we were drawing to a close and wanted to have enough time in our final session. I also told him that I did have a lot on my mind, but mainly it was just recapping some of the highlights of our past sessions. Bob seemed to more than understand where I was coming from and told me that he was always happy to hear clients say that they feel that they are drawing to a close; after all, closure is a good thing.

"So, how do you feel about conducting our last session via telephone?" Bob asked.

"I have no problem with it. I was the one who actually suggested it. We can always jump on a webinar if need be," I said.

"That's true," Bob said.

"Heck, Bob, this could turn out to be a new avenue of revenue growth for you," I said.

"That's not a half-bad idea, Michael. Why don't we get going and see how things work out, OK?" Bob asked.

I have to admit, it was kind of nice lying in bed getting psychoanalyzed while eating English muffins and watching the news in my boxers.

"Do you want to pick up where we left off?" Bob asked.

"Yeah, that's fine. If I'm correct, I believe we left off talking about my marriage and all the fun things that came with that," I said.

"Yeah, I think you may be selling yourself short a bit. After all, we did talk about quite a bit more than your marriage, so I hope that you're just abbreviating it for my sake," he said.

"No, you're absolutely correct, I was just abbreviating it and didn't mean to make light of it at all," I said. "Is it kind of odd for you, Bob, to be psychoanalyzing me without having me there in your office?" I asked.

"No, not really. This isn't the first time for me, so I'm a little used to it," Bob said. "Why, is there something I need to know?"

"No, not at all, I was just checking with you," I said. I found it kind of odd that Bob never made mention of the fact that I had not seen him in so long. I mean that literally years had gone by. I had been in touch with him on certain occasions, but I had not been into the office since the end of my marriage. I decided to ask Bob about this and why he hadn't mentioned that there had been such a large gap between sessions.

"Michael, I have to apologize to you if this is a sensitive subject, but I see a lot of people, and a lot of them simply drop off the map after only two or three sessions. I've also had a lot of people like you who may go years without seeing me but stay in touch either by phone or by e-mail. How does it make you feel now that I have explained the matter in detail?"

"Well, that's kinda what I expected, but I feel it's always better to ask than assume," I said.

I felt a little more relaxed than normal; I guess it must've been the fact that I knew that I had booked a double session and I wouldn't be pushed for time. I'm sure that my comfortable surroundings didn't hurt too much either. Bob's office had always made me feel comfortable, but I would've given anything to be able to stretch out on one of his leather couches. Getting up and stretching out when you're in a wheelchair, however, is pretty much impossible unless you have some serious help.

I told Bob that I had finally lost the use of my legs during my divorce. I guess it was the stress that finally overwhelmed me and made me take a seat so to speak. Before going into a wheelchair, I started out with a limp, and then began using a cane, and finally a walker. The limp, or what the doctors termed drop foot, started when I was living in Denver. I was like the Darwinian theory in reverse—de-evolution.

I was building a new home at the time near the foothills of the Rocky Mountains on a beautiful lot of land that was surrounded by nothing except an old horse farm for miles around. To watch the dark storm clouds of a winter's twilight blizzard roll down from the mountains and blanket the towns below under the bright moon's glow was like looking into the very core of God's creation. The juxtaposition of His creations could not be more well-defined; unfortunately, I wished I was more like the winter snowfalls.

"So at some point I'm assuming that you had to let work know about your condition once you had to start using a cane due to drop foot. Can you tell me about how that happened and how you worked your way through it?" Bob asked.

"Well, it must've been around the summer of 1995 because that's when my wife's mother and father came out to visit us for a week's vacation in Aspen. By the way, that was actually the first time that I had come to understand what all the jokes pertaining to mothers-in-law were about, except I wasn't laughing. My wife had planned a big white-water rafting trip down the Colorado River as one of our activities. The president of my company gave me permission to use one of our corporate condominiums, and boy, was it beautiful. Unfortunately for me, I only made it about a third of the way through the rafting trip before we ended up hitting some pretty hard white water where I was thrown out the raft and tore my ACL in my left knee.

"We ended up driving home earlier than planned as my knee had become quite swollen and difficult to walk on. When we got home, I ended up going straight to the ER due to the pain in my knee, and they told me that I had torn my ACL and actually fractured my tibia right below my knee, which was what was causing all of the pain and problems walking. They gave me a walking cast and a pair of crutches post-surgery, both of which I was supposed to use for a period of three months," I said.

"The best that I can remember, this is when the cascade of lies began. Believe me, it's true what they say about lying—one lie just leads to another. I guess that one of the engineers in our department had noticed that I was still using a cane after month number four, and apparently, she asked my friend Mike why, as ACL tears only took three to three and a half months to heal properly. I'll never forget the day that Mike came into my office, shut the door, and then proceeded to question me about what was really going on with my leg.

"My face must have been deep red when he asked me, because I could feel the heat rising off my face like an old steam radiator furnace. I had absolutely no time to even begin to dream up another lie, and I knew at that point that I had finally been caught in my own web of lies—it was over. I recall Mike's jaw hanging agape as I told him the true story and how long I had been battling to keep it a secret—close to two and a half years. I couldn't stop apologizing to him; after all, he was my best friend. Much to my surprise, Mike wasn't mad at all; he was just severely upset for me, and he also had the common sense to know that I could no longer go on telling the lie as people were starting to talk now and work needed to know.

"I received what I thought were two conflicting pieces of advice. My doctor told me that telling work about my MS was a personal decision, one that I needed to make on my own. Mike's opinion was that I needed to let work know immediately as my peers were apparently becoming concerned for my well-being. Mike and his fiancée at the time, Laura, graciously invited Michelle and I over for dinner that weekend so we had some time to sit around and talk openly about the matter. I guess you need to understand, Bob, that my number one concern was losing my job because I was no longer physically capable of performing all aspects of it (a large portion of my job was dedicated toward traveling). I think that Michelle also shared some of my concerns about being let go from my current position.

"In the end, however, I finally decided to talk with the president of our company and my boss, with the director of human resources acting as my liaison.

"It was very difficult, as I'm sure you can imagine, for me to tell my story, including the details leading up to me finally coming forward to them. I have to say that if you have never seen anyone in true shock before, they would have made a picture perfect portrait. Almost immediately after telling my side of the story, I thought I was going to be escorted out of the building, but our president just kept talking about how much they had failed me as an employee and that if one of their top guys was so scared about losing his job that he would not talk to management, how the rest of the group must have felt," I said.

"I cannot even begin to imagine how you must have felt and what you must have been going through. I mean, I know we've talked about this in broad strokes before but have never gotten down to this level of detail. I don't know what else to say but I'm sorry, Michael. I take it you didn't get fired, correct?" Bob asked.

Laughing, I said, "No, like I said, they were just really embarrassed, and I was really relieved."

"How about your divorce, Michael? Are you still having some problems?" Bob asked.

"I thought that I had sent you an e-mail regarding the fact that things were still not going too well," I said.

"You're correct. I'm sorry, you did send me an e-mail and told me that things weren't going too well," he said.

I sat quietly in my wheelchair for a moment before I reclined it into a more comfortable position. My electronic wheelchair was definitely the Cadillac of chairs. It had just about every function and feature you could imagine in a chair, and one of the most satisfying aspects was being able to recline it electronically with the touch of just the joystick. The nice part was that it took the pressure off of my buttocks and placed it directly onto my back, which was something that I found that I needed following my post-op surgery period. I broke from protocol for a moment and sent Bob some pictures as I wanted to show him the new wheelchair and the features on it.

"Yeah, I have a few of my patients who have wheel-chairs like that, but now that I look at it up close, they're not nearly as fancy as this one is. This is really pretty impressive, everything that it can do. Do you mind me asking how much it was?" Bob asked.

"No, not at all. If memory serves me right, it was twenty-four thousand five hundred dollars, of which I paid zero. Can you freaking believe that? Not having to pay a single penny toward my deductible. As luck would have it, I had already paid my deductible in full, and when they finally got off their lazy asses and got me my wheelchair—which they had been promis-ing for months on end—I didn't owe them a penny," I said.

"I guess it is true what they say: some things are well worth the wait," he said.

"Anyway, I apologize, what were we just talking about prior to the wheelchair…my divorce?" I asked.

"Yes, is your divorce still ongoing, or has it finally come to an end?" Bob asked.

"Well, I have to admit that after seven years of bick-ering and fighting, the divorce is finally wrapping up," I said. "We were married for a total span of twelve years, ten months, three weeks, and one day, including the time since I was physically served the divorce papers. I guess if there's any good to come out of it, we did beat the seven-year average."

Bob replied by saying how sorry he was to hear the bad news; I was still having a debate with myself as to whether or not my divorce was a bad thing or not. "I know that to you, it may make very little difference, but we therapists sometimes like to know who initiated the divorce and why," Bob said.

"Just sticking to the facts for now, Bob, but it was definitely her who wanted the divorce in the first place. I was completely caught off guard and not expecting it at all. It was like draining blood from a turnip, but I finally got her to admit that she simply could not handle dealing with the effects of multiple sclerosis. She sat in front of God, our parents, our families, and our friends and did nothing short of betraying all of us. I don't like going down this road too much as I am not her judge or executioner, and as filled with hate and rage I may feel at times, I beg God for the patience and the understanding to move on," I said.

There was silence on the phone. Bob must have been doing some daydreaming. Probably thinking of my ex-wife and what type of person it takes to leave some-one—check that, to leave your *spouse* in need. I went on to explain to Bob that my feelings of angst were far diminished from what they used to be. Those feelings had been replaced by sorrow; sorrow for my children and for all that they missed, essentially growing up without a father while their mother somehow tried to make up for her teenage years of Catholicism.

I told Bob that for the longest time, my two youngest children were actually afraid of me. As I started to grow older, they began to blame me for the divorce as it was obvious that she was directing them to me for questions that I simply did not have answers to—in essence, she was brainwashing them. "I should mention that she was finally directed by the court not to involve the children in any manners related to the divorce itself," I said. This ended up coming from the judge himself only after hiring a guardian ad litem (GAL) for the case who discovered that my ex-wife had, in fact, been doing all of the things that I claimed she was, which was mainly bad-mouthing me, telling the kids how bad a father I was, and so on. My heart was broken as well as my mind, and I ended up going into a deep depression for which I neither sought nor wanted any help.

"Did you ever contemplate suicide, Michael?" Bob asked.

I paused for what seemed like minutes before answering, staring at the wall in front of me as if waiting for the answer to pop out. I knew the answer, but it was a personal subject and one that obviously I didn't like to talk about. "Yes, countless times, but I obviously never acted on it. I never could come to harm myself," I responded.

"And how do you feel now?" Bob asked.

Again, I paused before answering Bob as tears streamed down my face. I knew that if I gave him an honest answer I might find myself being committed. I could not speak as I knew that the crackle in my voice would betray me. I held out for as long as I possibly could before Bob would demand an answer to his simple question. "I feel like I finally have some closure, even if it did come with great losses physically, mentally, and financially," I finally said.

There was a pause on the other end of the line, and I felt for a moment that maybe Bob did not believe my lie. I removed my glasses and wiped the tears from my eyes.

"I can only begin to imagine what you may still be going through, Michael, and I want you to know that I'm always here for you, OK?" he said.

"Thanks, Bob, I really appreciate your thoughts," I said.

"And your children, Michael? How are they doing right now? Have they come to see the truth in the matter, or do they still believe in an alternate reality so to speak?" Bob asked.

"From a parent's point of view, Bob, I can see that they are healed on the outside like a wound develops a scab, but it would not take much to scratch away that scab and expose bleeding flesh again. I also understand something that they don't right now and probably won't for quite some time: they lost out on so much of their own childhood simply due to the selfishness of their own mother who they thought was their best friend. Hell, for that matter, I lost out also. I lost so much time with my children that it's actually scary to think about. She stole them from me. She stole time from me. I don't know, Bob, maybe I'm different than other fathers. I happen to give a shit and that has made me the bad guy.

"The more I think about it and the more I care, the more it hurts. I'm well aware of what I've lost, and I'm also well aware of the fact that I'll never gain it back. There is simply nothing that I can do or say now that would help the matter any. The only thing that I can do is tell them how much I love them every chance that I get," I said.

"I'm tired, Bob. I'm tired of talking and rehashing the past. Give yourself a scorecard and tell me on a ranking from zero to ten, with zero being the worst, if you feel you have been able to help me throughout these years," I said.

"Hmm, I've certainly never been asked to do an evaluation of myself right in front of one of my own clients—interesting. Did you just come up with this on your own, Michael?" Bob responded.

"Yes, yes, I just now came up with this little self-evaluation. Everybody always wants to evaluate me, so for once, I'd like to see a therapist evaluate themselves," I said.

"OK, that's fair. If I had to evaluate myself right now, I would give myself a score of seven," he said. "Now you know I'm not going to let you get off the hook that quick, Michael, I'd like to personally know what score you would give me."

"Well, I have to admit that I've been thinking about this for some time now, and as far as the score goes, I would give you the same, or maybe a little higher—let's just call it a seven point five," I said. "Bob, all joking aside, I have a serious issue that I'd like to discuss with you."

"Sure, Michael, what's going on?" he asked.

I was sitting at my kitchen table in my wheelchair, working on my computer when I decided to talk to Bob about this latest issue. I was on speakerphone, and

I was anxious. This was one of those issues that had been placed inside the lockbox in my head and the key thrown away. I'd tried desperately to just live in the moment and forget about it, but something came up and I just couldn't let go.

"Michael, you still on the line? Are you OK? Michael, you're going to have to give me an answer soon, or I'm going to have to make a phone call, OK?" Bob asked.

"Bob, do you remember me telling you about how I had to stay in a nursing home during part of my five-month recovery?" I asked.

"Sure, of course I do. Those places can be pretty rough. Did something happen to you while you were there?" he asked.

"No…well, yes, something did happen, but that's kinda beside the point," I said. "I don't think I've ever talked to you about my living arrangements and my caretaker, have I?" I asked.

"Well, you did mention that your mother was your caretaker and had been since, I believe, your separation from your wife," Bob said.

"That's right—I remember now that we did briefly talk about it, but I'd like to put a bow on that issue if you will and ask you for some extended help," I said.

"Sure, sure, tell me what's going on," he said.

"Well, to complete my story, I don't know how much you know about MS patients, but a large majority of them need what's called a caretaker. In my case, it's especially true because of my paraplegia and the fact that there are just certain things that there's no way I can to do without someone's help, like getting in and out of my bed and transferring to and from my wheelchair. Since my return home and during my further recuperation, my father fell and had to have an operation on his spinal column to repair a fracture in one of his vertebra.

"Long story short, he awoke from surgery with less-than-expected results. While the vertebra was repaired, he lost the function of his legs and is also now a paraplegic bound to a wheelchair. Since my mother was the only person taking care of both of us, I had to hire a CNA to help bathe me and get me out of bed and into the wheelchair every morning. Regardless of all this, I can see that my mother is near her breaking point, so I'm concerned that all of us may wind up in nursing homes, which my father and I simply will not do."

"So if I understand your situation correctly, you have no other family besides your mother and father, and then obviously your younger kids. Is that correct?" Bob asked.

"That's correct. So I hope I'm making some sense to you here, but by main concern is what is going to happen to me when my parents pass," I said. "After living in that one nursing home for over a month, I can tell you that there is no way that I would go back to one of those hellholes again, and trust me, they're all the same. I hate to say it, but when I lose my parents, I lose my life. Does any of this make sense?" I asked.

"Yeah, Michael, it makes perfect sense, and I have to be honest with you here by telling you that you put me in quite a conundrum," Bob said. "Nursing homes and long-term care are simply not within my wheelhouse. Now, with that said, I'm sure that I can work with you to try to find some long-term care that better meets your needs or expectations."

"I appreciate it, Bob, I really do, but you also have to understand how long I've already been looking and how much research I've already been doing on this subject matter. Let me just tell you that anything that even comes close to interesting is so far out of my price range that I can only laugh at it. Listen to me carefully; I truly feel that when my parents' lives are over, so is mine. I don't mean to be rude, Bob, but I just don't want you spinning your wheels as I can tell you that no matter what you say, short of a miracle, it will make no difference with me," I said.

"Point taken, Michael, but I have to ask you if you would allow me some more time to do some research on my own," Bob said.

Silence—nothing but awkward silence. "You can do what you want, but I'm telling you right now that you're just spinning your wheels. Game over!" I said.

That was the last conversation that I had with Bob, and while it was good getting things off my chest, we really didn't get too much accomplished, at least not from my point of view.

A Farewell to Kings

When did I finally decide to wake up? The truth of the matter is that I have been wide awake this entire time. I have not been asleep at my post, I have not abandoned you, and I have never ignored you. If this is what you believe, you have taken me for a fool. I have, however, been depleted of my life force by the endless, mind-numbing pain and problems that this disease has seemingly forever plagued me with. I have spent more than half my life consumed by something that I can neither control nor come to terms with; after twenty-five years, I still lack understanding. By my own choosing, this is a burden that I have attempted to carry alone for too long. It is who I am; I am a heavyweight fighter who should have retired years ago, but the term *retire* is not in my vocabulary.

I am guilty of closing the blinds on those around me—my family, my friends. I have let endless hours, days, and years slowly slip through my fingers like sand, without recourse. I have let go of my end of the rope while you were struggling to hold the other, and for this act alone, I am deeply sorry.

What are you sorry for? I have asked God for forgiveness. He is always there, always willing to forgive; I realize now that the same cannot be said of you, but I do not judge you; it is not my place. With the time that He has so generously granted me, I will spend it by your sides, trying my best to reconcile with all the time lost. Always remember that my love for each of you is endless and will last forever, regardless of the outcome that may one day come to bear its full weight on me.

I find it harder to run this marathon; time seemingly increases in speed with my age. My only goal is to finish the race with my children by my side. Time seems to run exponentially now where once it was linear.

I feel myself diverging further and further away from my children now. The physical pain is easier to deal with than the pain within my heart; I must make every day count. I am a star at twilight circling a massive black hole. My fate lies ahead of me and is predetermined. I feel my once brightly shining light fading now, shredded and devoured by the machine that lies ahead on the horizon, yet all I can think about are my precious children, my gifts from God. My love for them is endless and knows no bounds; it is absolute and forever. Am I, like so many others, guilty of wasting one of God's most precious gifts?

As I reflect on my life to date, I must realize that I have not squandered this gift. I have used it to accomplish the goals that I set into motion early in life and that helped me to become the man I am today. Others are not so fortunate, and this fact should not be lost on you. Yes, I am grateful for the time that I have been given and for what I have chosen to do with it. I believe that somehow time is a universal gift to be used wisely. If it were not, our lifespan would be indefinite, and time would have no true meaning for us. I believe that as we grow older, most of us, and especially those who have been diagnosed with a terminal disease, wish for just a few more precious moments with our families.

Time seems to stretch like an endless fiber pulled from a spool of unknown diameter far out into the darkness of infinity. Our lives lie along this length of fiber. It is here where life begins and ends. In between, we meet one another, we get married, we have children, and we have grandchildren. We are here for the memories of our own children, to give them hope.

What is the last thing that I will see moments prior to my death? I pray that the answer is my family. I pray also that they are the first thing that I see when I reawaken to a new and glorious day as created and promised by God Almighty.

Hang on to every moment you have, share your immense propensity for love with your family, and tell them how much you love them every opportunity you get; tomorrow may never come. Squander not a single moment. Do not abandon those who seek your love, your guidance, and your attention. March toward the darkness wherever possible, shine your light brightly, and fear not, for He is with us all.

I despise the loneliness, the darkness. Once again, I feel the tears well up in my eyes, not out of self-pity but from my love for each of you. I feel them stream down my face. I am tired now, tired of tasting the bitter salt of these tears of chronic depression. I am tired of thinking of what these tears represent for me and my family. For nearly twenty-five years, I have battled. I believed, I hoped, I wished for a cure, a miracle, anything that would allow me to step out of this chair and walk hand in hand with each of you. I cannot hold or hug my children in the manner in which my heart so desperately desires; I know I never will.

Is this how I will be judged? Is this how I should be judged? My heart tells me otherwise; my heart tells me that I am judged by my children and by my family, for who I am and what I do. Of this, I have no doubt. When people look at me and inquire why I am in a wheelchair, I stare them straight in the eyes and tell them that I have multiple sclerosis. When they inevitably next tell me how sorry they are, I tell them not to be for I would not have turned out to be the man I am today. Approach life this way, my children. Tackle it head on. Grab the proverbial bull by the horns and wrestle it to the ground. The only thing that you cannot accomplish is what your mind tells you.

My Faceless Enemy

Depression is my faceless enemy;
I turn to look back but instead
find it one step ahead of me.
Thoughts of suicide have pervad-
ed my mind and left me empty.
Questions I have, answers I
don't; the tears are plenty.
I'll just let my emotions go; I'll try
hard to clear my head and fly.
Fly, fly away—is it easier to just say good-bye?

Mistakes that I have been blamed
for alter my mood.
Just let me, please, talk to you.
We talk; however, it's depres-
sion that whispers over all of us.
This is its secret over me.
To be as silent as can be,, open
your ears, please listen to me.
Monsters do exist, but they don't
hide in closets or under beds.
They hide deep in our heads.
Ignore a call for help at your own peril.
Best friends don't talk over each oth-
er; they listen. Be careful.
I ask each of you for one of your
greatest gifts—time.
Be at rest now, be quiet now, muffle
the noises, and take a look around.
Learn to read between the lines.
Shine your bright and loving light into the dark-
ness, walk the lonely to help, and be not afraid.
Help them to live another day.
—Michael